T0395426

VOLUME ONE HUNDRED AND SIXTY FIVE

ADVANCES IN
IMMUNOLOGY

Advances in DNA and
mRNA-Based Strategies for Cancer
Immunotherapy: Part A

ASSOCIATE EDITORS

Fritz Melchers
University of Basel, Basel, Switzerland

Chen Dong
Shanghai Jiaotong University School of Medicine,
Tsinghua University School of Medicine

Hao Wu
Boston Children's Hospital, Harvard Medical School

VOLUME ONE HUNDRED AND SIXTY FIVE

ADVANCES IN
IMMUNOLOGY

Advances in DNA and mRNA-Based Strategies for Cancer Immunotherapy: Part A

Edited by

ARUN KUMAR SINGH

Department of Pharmacy, Vivekananda Global University, Jaipur, Rajasthan, India

NEERAJ MISHRA

Professor and Head of Department, Amity Institute of Pharmacy, Amity University, Gwalior, Madhya Pradesh, India

SUMEL ASHIQUE

Department of Pharmaceutical Technology, Bharat Technology, Uluberia, West Bengal, India

PRANAV KUMAR PRABHAKAR

Department of Biotechnology, School of Engineering and Technology, Nagaland University, Meriema, Kohima, Nagaland, India

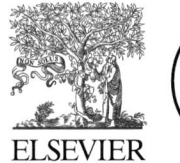

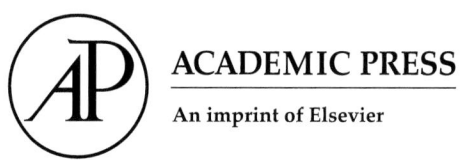

ACADEMIC PRESS

An imprint of Elsevier

Academic Press is an imprint of Elsevier
125 London Wall, London, EC2Y 5AS, United Kingdom
50 Hampshire Street, 5th Floor, Cambridge, MA 02139, United States

First edition 2025

Notices
Knowledge and best practice in this field are constantly changing. As new research and experience broaden our understanding, changes in research methods, professional practices, or medical treatment may become necessary.

Practitioners and researchers must always rely on their own experience and knowledge in evaluating and using any information, methods, compounds, or experiments described herein. In using such information or methods they should be mindful of their own safety and the safety of others, including parties for whom they have a professional responsibility.

To the fullest extent of the law, neither the Publisher nor the authors, contributors, or editors, assume any liability for any injury and/or damage to persons or property as a matter of products liability, negligence or otherwise, or from any use or operation of any methods, products, instructions, or ideas contained in the material herein.

ISBN: 978-0-443-34495-4
ISSN: 0065-2776

For information on all Academic Press publications
visit our website at https://www.elsevier.com/books-and-journals

Publisher: Zoe Kruze
Acquisitions Editor: Leticia Lima
Editorial Project Manager: Palash Sharma
Production Project Manager: Sujatha Thirugnana Sambandam
Cover Designer: Bakyalakshmi S

Typeset by MPS Limited, India

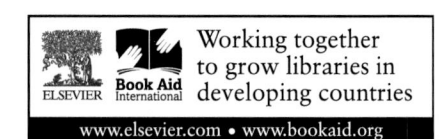

Working together
to grow libraries in
developing countries

www.elsevier.com • www.bookaid.org

Contents

5. mRNA-based cancer vaccines: A novel approach to melanoma treatment   **117**

Pranav Kumar Prabhakar, Tarun Kumar Upadhyay, and Sanjeev Kumar Sahu

6. Therapeutic mRNAs for cancer immunotherapy: From structure to delivery   163

Monika Vishwakarma, Wasim Akram, and Tanweer Haider

Contributors

Garima
M.M College of Pharmacy, Maharishi Markandeshwar (Deemed to be University), Mullana-Ambala, Haryana, India

Jagriti
Department of Biochemistry, All India Institute of Medical Sciences, Gorakhpur, Uttar Pradesh, India

Wasim Akram
Amity Institute of Pharmacy, Amity University Madhya Pradesh, Gwalior, Madhya Pradesh, India

Sumel Ashique
Department of Pharmaceutical Technology, Bharat Technology, Uluberia, West Bengal, India

Sombuddha Biswas
Department of Preventive and Social Medicine (Public Health), JIPMER Puducherry, India

Pramila Chaubey
Department of Pharmaceutics, College of Pharmacy, Shaqra University, Shaqra, Kingdom of Saudi Arabia

Isha Chawla
M.M College of Pharmacy, Maharishi Markandeshwar (Deemed to be University), Mullana-Ambala, Haryana, India

Meenakshi Dhanawat
Amity Institute of Pharmacy, Amity University Haryana, Amity Education Valley, Panchgaon, Manesar, Gurugram, Haryana, India

Iman Ehsan
Research Associate, National Institute of Pharmaceutical Education and Research, Kolkata, West Bengal, India

Karan Goel
M.M College of Pharmacy, Maharishi Markandeshwar (Deemed to be University), Mullana-Ambala, Haryana, India

Tanweer Haider
Gyan Vihar School of Pharmacy, Suresh Gyan Vihar University, Jaipur, Rajasthan, India

Anas Islam
Faculty of Pharmacy, Integral University, Lucknow, Uttar Pradesh, India

Naheed Mojgani
Biotechnology Department, Razi vaccine and serum Research Institute, Agricultural Research, Education and Extension Organization, Karaj, Iran

Pranav Kumar Prabhakar
Department of Biotechnology, School of Engineering and Technology, Nagaland University, Meriema, Kohima, Nagaland, India

Sanjeev Kumar Sahu
School of Pharmaceutical Sciences, Lovely Professional University, Phagwara, Punjab, India

Aniruddha Sen
Department of Biochemistry, All India Institute of Medical Sciences, Gorakhpur, Uttar Pradesh, India

Arun Kumar Singh
Department of Pharmacy, Vivekananda Global University, Jaipur, Rajasthan, India

Vijay Singh
Department of Biochemistry, All India Institute of Medical Sciences, Gorakhpur, Uttar Pradesh, India

Tarun Kumar Upadhyay
Parul Institute of Applied Sciences & Research and Development Cell, Parul University, Vadodara, Gujarat, India

Monika Vishwakarma
Department of Pharmaceutical Sciences, Doctor Harisingh Gour University, Sagar, Madhya Pradesh; Faculty of Pharmacy, Kalinga University, Naya Raipur, Chhattisgarh, India

Kashish Wilson
M.M College of Pharmacy, Maharishi Markandeshwar (Deemed to be University), Mullana-Ambala, Haryana, India

DNA and mRNA vaccines: Significant therapeutic approach against cancer management

Aniruddha Sen[a], Vijay Singh[a], Sumel Ashique[b,*] (iD), Jagriti[a], Sombuddha Biswas[c], Anas Islam[d], Iman Ehsan[e], and Naheed Mojgani[f]

[a]Department of Biochemistry, All India Institute of Medical Sciences, Gorakhpur, Uttar Pradesh, India
[b]Department of Pharmaceutical Technology, Bharat Technology, Uluberia, West Bengal, India
[c]Department of Preventive and Social Medicine (Public Health), JIPMER Puducherry, India
[d]Faculty of Pharmacy, Integral University, Lucknow, Uttar Pradesh, India
[e]Research Associate, National Institute of Pharmaceutical Education and Research, Kolkata, West Bengal, India
[f]Biotechnology Department, Razi vaccine and serum Research Institute, Agricultural Research, Education and Extension Organization, Karaj, Iran
*Corresponding author e-mail address: ashiquesumel007@gmail.com

Contents

Advances in Immunology, Volume 165
ISSN 0065-2776, https://doi.org/10.1016/bs.ai.2024.10.007

Abstract

Cancer's complex nature and personal variety make it among the toughest cancers to conquer. Innovative treatment strategies can be achieved through new biotechnology developments. DNA and mRNA vaccinations deliver an opportunity to take a new path for cancer. The ways in which DNA and mRNA vaccinations generate immune reactions that specifically focus on cancer cells are discussed in this section. This chapter focuses on the development and creation of these vaccines. We will focus on the latest research that proves the effectiveness of these vaccines and their safety over different types of cancer. Also, we discuss the technological and biological barriers in the process of vaccine development that hinder the development of these vaccines, such as the stability of delivery methods and a patient-specific design for vaccines. DNA and mRNA vaccinations are an important therapeutic approach against cancer with genetic information. They offer an opportunity for the future to develop tailored as well as more efficient treatment options.

1. Introduction

Cancer is among the most challenging cancers to fight, mostly because of its variety and complexity. Different types of cancer have distinct characteristics that render an approach that is universally applicable ineffective. The heterogeneity of tumors, in which various cells in the same tumor display distinct phenotypic and genetic profiles can make treatment more difficult (Chakraborty & Rahman, 2012a). Additionally, conventional medicines such as chemotherapy and radiation can trigger cancer cells to develop resistance and make treatment challenges worse (Zugazagoitia et al., 2016). A further issue is the late diagnosis since many malignancies develop at advanced levels where there are a limited number of inadequate treatment options (Garg et al., 2023). Additionally, the negative side effects of conventional treatment for cancer could adversely impact the patient's health and quality of life. It may cause patients to stop the treatment. Treatments are usually focused on healthy as well as cancerous tissue, which can produce a multitude of negative outcomes (Zugazagoitia et al., 2016; Schilsky et al., 2010). It is imperative to devise less-invasive and targeted treatments that can energetically eradicate cancer cells while not affecting healthy tissues. Immunotherapy attacking the tumor using our own immune system body to detect and destroy the cancerous cells has made the treatment of cancer patient to change. Immunotherapies boost the immune system's capability to detect cancer and fight it while other treatments consider their focus within cancer cells only. This approach led to the development of a number of promising treatments including those that are based on adoption based cell transplants, checkpoint inhibitors and monoclonal antibodies (Kumar et al., 2021). For example, the monoclonal antibodies have been developed to be glued to specific antigens present on the outer shell of cancerous cells, thus pointing their immune system as an enemy. On the other hand, checkpoint inhibitors inhibit antibodies that prevent immune response that causes T cells to attack cancerous cell lines (Galmarini, 2020). Adoptive-cell transfer is patients' infusion with immune cells that pre-treated or regenerated outside of the organism to increase their anti-tumor activity (Debela et al., 2021).

In many cases these treatments are paying off much more now than before as they offer the cancer patients a chance to try something different where ordinary Therapy has not yielded. There are still issues, for example, immunogenicity adverse reactions and the variations in patients' profile remain problems. This suggests that one needs to continue searching for more substantiation and to refine methods in an attempt to enhance the efficacy of immune therapy (Feeley et al., 2014). This treatment method which includes DNA and m RNA some of the genetic vaccines that have been used in treatment of cancer is thus a breakthrough. TAAs implies tumor associated antigens which are the genes transported in the body by these vaccines. They triggered the formation in the immune system towards the development of a special tool to eliminate cancerous cell bearing Antigens (Foulkes and Sharpless, 2021). It has been found that a vast majority of DNA vaccines employ the plasmids that carry genes which would help in the manufacturing of TAAs. These plasmids are then introduced into the body and the cells actively uptake the DNA and begin to produce the antigen that triggers Immune response. On the other hand, it is conveyed by the mRNA-based vaccine or also known as messenger RNA or mRNA for short and stands for deoxyribonucleic acid. It then invades the cell of the host where the mRNA of the cell is used to produce antigen which as a result triggers an immune response (Yuzhalin, 2024). Another major advantage is that genetic vaccines provide highly specific targeted immune response, which, most likely, means fewer 'side bad effects' than standard treatments. They can also be rapidly developed and manufactured that makes it possible for them to be tailored for different kinds of cancers and even individual genetic markers for the patient (Zugazagoitia et al., 2016; Chakraborty & Rahman, 2012). The major advancement so far in cancer treatment has been experienced through the recent clinical trials that have shown the effectiveness and safety of the mRNA and DNA vaccines against the various forms of cancer (Dede et al., 2023; Ventola, 2017). Despite the potential positives of developing genetic vaccines, there are challenges that come with it including; challenges in delivering the genetic material, challenges that arise in the stability of the material and lastly, the challenge of patient variability. For the DNA and mRNA vaccines to offer a comprehensive opportunity in cancer treatments, more studies are focused on trying to overcome these challenges (Schilsky et al., 2010).

2. Principles of DNA and mRNA vaccines

Tumor-associated antigens can be genetically inserted into a patient's own cells by the use of mRNA and DNA vaccines in order to stimulate an immune response against cancerous cells. DNA vaccines introduces TAA genes in to host cells through plasmids where it is converted into an mRNA after being transduced. If these proteins are detected on cells' surfaces and cytotoxic lymphocytes (CTLs) are activated which allows them to fight and eliminate cancerous cells. Through the delivery of synthetic mRNA inside lipid nanoparticles directly into host cells MRNA-based vaccines can stimulate an immune reaction by activating CTLs. In this case, the mRNA gets converted into TAAs. Both approaches aim to make use of the immune system to detect and eradicate cancerous cells. DNA vaccines are well-known for their long-lasting durability and immune system, while mRNA vaccinations provide rapid development as well as powerful immune reactions (Kutzler and Weiner, 2008; Pardi et al., 2018).

2.1 Basic mechanisms

DNA vaccines are created through the introduction of a plasmid inside host cells which has the DNA sequence codifying for the antigen targeted. The cells take in this virus and transport it to the nucleus in which the messenger transcript (mRNA) generated by the host's cells converts DNA. Within the cytoplasm, an antigenic protein is then made by converting the messenger RNA. Major Histocompatibility Complex (MHC) cells process and display the antigen that they have created at the cell's surface, stimulating cellular and humoral immune reactions. It basically "trains" the immune system to recognize and fight the virus if it's encountered in the future (Liu, 2019; Cui, 2005).

The mechanism that works with mRNA-based vaccines is through directly delivering synthesized mRNA molecules that code for the antigen targeted into the cells of the host. To stop the deterioration process and help in cellular metabolism, the MRNA molecules are encased in the form of lipid nanoparticles. The targeted protein is created when the mRNA is introduced into the cells of the host through the cell's ribosomes. After the processing process, the produced protein antigen can be seen on the surface of cells through MHC molecules. This triggers an immune reaction. The reaction outcome in the formation of specific antibodies as well as T-cell activation. These cells protect against the possibility of infection from the pathogen with the same antigen soon (Fig. 1) (Liu, 2019; Gote et al., 2023).

2.1.1 Transcription and translation dynamics

The fundamental principles of molecular biology–transcription and translation are involved in the core mechanisms of DNA and mRNA vaccines. Plasmid DNA is the genetic blueprint of a particular antigen that is used in DNA-based vaccines. The DNA plasmid is taken into cells following its introduction into the body. This is usually done together with electroporation or vectors that are viral. The process of transcription is by that the plasmid DNA can be transformed into messenger (mRNA) after it has been placed in the nucleus of the cell (Pilkington et al., 2021).

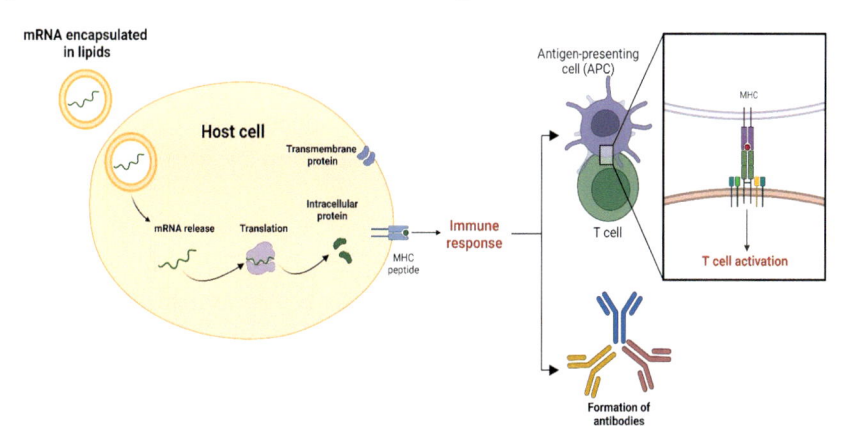

Fig. 1 This figure illustrates the detailed cellular process from the entry of mRNA encapsulated in lipid nanoparticles to the elicitation of an immune response through antigen presentation and T cell activation.

Injecting the mRNA directly into the cytoplasm of the host cell mRNA vaccines bypass the transcription phase. Nanoparticles of Lipid (LNPs) contain the microRNAs, which are synthesized in vitro and encode the antigen of interest, thereby shielding it from degradation while also promoting cell uptake (Gote et al., 2023). After the mRNA reaches the cell's cytoplasm then ribosomes turn it into a targeted protein. It is transformed before being evident on the surface of the cell (Föhse et al., 2023a).

The antibodies must be identified so that the immune system can become active in the near future. Antigens appear in Major Histocompatibility (MHC) molecules as they are processed by the cells' normal processes. The immune system's adaptive as well as innate response is based on the appearance of these molecules (Heine et al., 2021).

2.1.2 Immune system activation

Many processes play a role in activating the immune system through the mRNA and DNA vaccines that ultimately lead to a strong and specific immune response. Antigen-presenting cells (APCs) like dendritic cells, can detect the antigen present from DNA vaccines once they are produced and displayed on cells' surfaces. They migrate to the lymph nodes of the body, they add T cells with the antigen that triggers the adaptive immune reaction (Verbeke et al., 2022).

Like this, the mRNA-based vaccines trigger powerful immune responses through antigens encoded. MHC molecules enable the antigens to be exhibited on cells' surfaces following conversion of the mRNA to the form of a protein. Then, it is processed. Helper T-cells get stimulated by this display, and the helper T-cells stimulate B-cells and cytotoxic cells. B-cells produce antibodies to neutralize the antigen. Cytotoxic T-cells are capable of killing cancer cells that express antigens by itself (Miao et al., 2021; Rosa et al., 2021).

In addition, because they recognize the molecules through pattern recognition receptors (PRRs) like TLRs (TLRs) These mRNA-based vaccines may boost the innate immune systems. Due to this recognition types I interferons as well as other cytokines are created that increase the immunity system overall (Debela et al., 2021). Since mRNA-based vaccines both activate the adaptive and innate immune systems, they have been extremely effective in stimulating an all-encompassing immune response to cancerous cell lines (Wang et al., 2023a).

2.2 Design and construction

2.2.1 Plasmid DNA vaccines

Within the world of genetic vaccines and plasmid DNA vaccination, these vaccines are an innovative and flexible direction. The procedure of making these vaccines begins with the selection of the appropriate antigen genes that are then put into plasmid carriers. These small, circular DNA vectors are ideal for carrying genetic material since they can reproduce by themselves inside the bacterial cell (Pandya et al., 2023; Gomez et al., 2022). A boost in the gene expression of the recombinant DNA in bacteria, the incorporation of the gene in the plasmid vector, and the cloning and identification of an antigen-specific gene are essential actions to produce an able-bodied plasmid DNA vaccine. To ensure that there is a high level of expression in the host cell the antigen genes are copied into a plasmid and are then put under the direction of a powerful promoter. The PCMV promoter is widely known and broadly used promoter because of its ubiquity and high activity in the mammalian cells (Cui, 2005; Porter & Raviprakash, 2017). Polyadenylation and introns are other features of the plasmid that frequently raise its stability as well as the performance of the mRNA transcription. The plasmid DNA gets created and amplified by bacteria in their cells after which it is purified for use to create a vaccine. Host cells take in the plasmid DNA when it has been administered, which allows it to get into the nucleus to undergo the process of mRNA transcription. The targeted antigen then gets created by translation of the mRNA before being exposed on the cell's surface, triggering an immune reaction (Przybylowski et al., 2007; Takada et al., 2020). The process stimulates cell and humoral immunity by mimicking natural disease. The process stimulates cell and humoral immunity by mimicking natural disease. Plasmid DNA vaccinations provide the advantage of creating long-lasting immune responses, with a lower risk of insertional mutagenesis or infection. Additionally, plasmid DNA-based vaccines are easily made for targeting cancer antigens, or new infections and they're very easy to create (Liu, 2019). However, there are many issues to solve, including efficient transport of target cells, especially in vivo, and the need for powerful adjuvants that boost the immune system. They are also research subjects (Sakib et al., 2020).

2.2.2 mRNA vaccine platforms

mRNA vaccines are attracting enough interest because of their flexibility, speedy development time, and high immunogenicity. The method of generating molecular mRNAs that contain the targeted antigen is referred to as mRNA design. Most often the process of in the in vitro process (IVT) can be used to produce these mRNAs by with a DNA-based template that includes all the necessary components to translate and transcription (Sayour et al., 2024).

The initial step to make the mRNA-based vaccines is to design a DNA template containing the antigen's coded sequence which is then surrounded by regulatory parts like that of poly(A) tail the 5 cap structure, and the areas that are not translated (UTRs). It is believed that the poly(A) tail enhances the durability of the mRNA within the cytoplasm. The $5'$ cap structure as well as UTRs are crucial to the stability and efficiency of translation of the mRNA (Miao et al., 2021; Li et al., 2023).

In order to create mRNA, DNA templates are created followed by IVT. Then, in order to stop the mRNA from degrading, and to allow the mRNAs to be absorbed by the cells of the host, it is improved and placed into the lipid nanoparticles (LNPs) (Pilkington et al., 2021). Since LNPs can bind to cell membranes and encapsulate the mRNA, allowing it to be absorbed into the cytoplasm, to be transformed into an antigen They are particularly efficient in the delivery of mRNA into cells. The organelles of the cells of the host then translate the mRNA into the targeted antigen. Following processing the antigen, is exposed to the cells on the surface. There it is the ability to activate an immune response (Santoro et al., 2018). Innate immune responses can be stimulated by this process which can also stimulate B and T cells. Pattern recognition receptors (PRRs) recognize the transcript (Heine et al., 2021).

mRNA-mediated vaccines impart many benefits. One of them is their rapid response to new infections and changes in cancer. They may be modified to code for several antigens improving their effectiveness. Additionally, they are not integrated into the genome of the host which reduces the chance of mutations that are insertional (Verbeke et al., 2022; Föhse et al., 2023b). Yet, the efficacy of the mRNA-based vaccination systems is dependent upon the stability and longevity of mRNA as well as how effective the methods of delivery (Pardi et al., 2018; Zhang et al., 2019).

2.3 Advantages of traditional approaches

Table 1 offers a thorough analysis of the major aspects, differences as well as challenges of DNA and mRNA vaccines with a focus on their distinct ways of delivery, as well as other crucial elements.

Table 1 Key differences, advantages, and challenges of DNA and mRNA vaccines.

Feature	DNA vaccines	mRNA vaccines
Mechanism of Action	Introduces plasmid DNA encoding antigens; DNA is transcribed into mRNA, which is then translated into protein antigens.	Delivers synthetic mRNA encoding antigens directly into the cytoplasm for translation into protein antigens.
Delivery Method	Plasmid vectors, often with electroporation or viral vectors.	Lipid nanoparticles (LNPs) encapsulation.
Development Speed	Relatively rapid due to synthetic processes but slower than mRNA.	Very rapid; exemplified by COVID-19 vaccine development.
Stability	Generally, more stable at higher temperatures.	Requires cold-chain logistics, often ultra-low temperatures.
Immune Response	Activates both humoral and cellular immunity; noted for stability and long-term immunity.	Activates both humoral and cellular immunity; noted for strong and rapid immune responses.
Manufacturing Complexity	Complex but well-understood; scalable with bacterial amplification.	Requires sophisticated facilities for RNA synthesis and LNP formulation.
Side Effects	Typically mild to moderate; long-term data available.	Typically mild to moderate; recent extensive safety data from COVID-19 vaccinations.
Challenges	Efficient delivery to target cells, need for potent adjuvants.	Stability of mRNA, efficient delivery systems, cold-chain logistics.
Clinical Trials	Demonstrated efficacy in several cancers; ongoing research to enhance immunogenicity.	Proven efficacy in COVID-19, promising results in cancer trials, ongoing research.
Cost	Generally lower production costs; established production methods.	Higher production costs due to advanced technology requirements.

2.3.1 Specificity and precision

With regards to the degree of particularity and accuracy in terms of specificity and precision, DNA and MRNA vaccines add significant advantages over traditional vaccines. Traditional vaccinations typically employ microorganisms inhibited or weakened to stimulate an immune reaction. The result can be negative effects and non-specific immune activation. But the vaccinations based upon DNA and mRNA can be used to create specific antigens which specifically targeted to trigger specific responses to the immune response (S. Venishaa et al., 2024). The ability of these vaccines to utilize genes to produce antibodies inside the host cell accounts for the accuracy. MRNA vaccines, like are engineered to contain precisely the sequence needed to produce a targeted antigen protein. Once the cell is in contact and being transformed into a protein which appears on the surface of cells and causes a powerful and targeted immune response (Verbeke et al., 2022; Sayour et al., 2024). To ensure only relevant antigens are created the strategy minimizes the risk of developing unexpected immune reactions and increases the efficacy of the vaccine. Also, the plasmid vectors can be utilized in DNA vaccines to deliver antigen-coding DNA into host cells. By utilizing powerful promoters and other regulators that raise the transcription of genes and translate the plasmids are designed to maximize the expression of antigens. The production of high levels of antigen is followed, which enhances and enhances the immune response (Lorentzen et al., 2022). Multiple epitopes may be contained in these vaccines due to their genetically engineered structures and could raise the specificity of the immune system as well as its range (Rahman et al., 2021a).

2.3.2 Rapid development cycles

This, therefore, makes the DNA and mRNA vaccines developed relatively faster than other methods, making this a major advantage. Conventional techniques of developing vaccines contain several tedious procedures which may require one or two years for instance, cultivation, inactivation and purification of the pathogens. However, because other vaccines including DNA and mRNA vaccines are artificial process and genetic patterns then their development time is much shorter (Liu, 2019; Föhse et al., 2023b). Some of the IVT methods which are utilized in this instance may assist in lowering the time which is taken to develop the MRNA vaccines. If the gene sequence of the target antigen is well established then it can be quickly translated into a formulated mRNA format. The use of this technique for making synthetic vaccines can offer the chance of a quick change and enhancement of the offering of a vaccine (Chaudhary et al., 2021). Also, unlike the traditional vaccines, no cell culture is used in the creation of the mRNA vaccines hence increasing easy and on the time taken to produce vaccines in large quantity (Borzova, 2024). To DNA vaccinations it is profitable to open the fast duplication and amplify of the antigen-coding DNA by the aid of the plasmids of bacteria. It can be easily amplified for production hence allowing for fast production of doses of vaccination (Przybylowski et al., 2007). Other backbones that maybe used include other backbones for plasmids that are likewise enhanced and also other molecular biological methods that have been confirmed may as well be used to foster the enhancement of the process. This means that the reaction to newly discovered infections and the spread of cancer among other diseases do not go out of control easily (Cui, 2005; Porter & Raviprakash, 2017).

In the COVID-19 epidemic, the rapid development phases of DNA as well as the mRNA vaccines were particularly evident. Within the first year after the outbreak, the mRNA vaccines were created, tested, and cleared for use in situations of emergency (Hani et al., 2023). The speed is unheard of and highlights the ability of these platforms to resolve quickly emerging cancer-related mutations as well as public health crises.

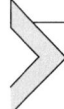

3. Development of DNA vaccines

3.1 Technological foundations

3.1.1 Synthetic techniques

The creation of precise DNA plasmid which contains antigen-coding sequences can be achieved with sophisticated techniques for synthetics that are essential for developing the development of DNA vaccines. Sequences of genetics that can be personalized are employed to create synthesized DNA to ensure that the created vaccines effectively trigger an immune response against specific cancers or antigens. Gene synthesis is among the main methods used to aid in creating the development of DNA-based vaccinations. The method lets DNA molecules to be created manually using nucleotides. The target gene is by the antigen that was initially identified, and later designed. it is synthesized using automatized oligonucleotide assemblies. This method allows the introduction of codon optimization that increases the amount of antigen expressed within human cells, by choosing codons that the host's translational apparatus can recognize (David et al., 2021; Wilson et al., 2021).

In addition, the use of modern molecular cloning procedures makes it easier to create the creation of synthetic DNA-based vaccines. Following synthesis then the desired DNA is placed into a plasmid carrying. The gene is transferred via this vector into cells of the host to produce within them. In the process of cloning ligases and restriction enzymes, are typically used to introduce genes into plasmids in specific locations, and to warrant that the gene is properly positioned and is surrounded by regulatory elements such as boosters and promoters (Matthews et al., 2022; Macheret & Halazonetis, 2015).

Beyond the standard methods and methods, the development of the CRISPR-Cas9-mediated cloning process and Gibson assembly have led to the creation of innovative technologies that deliver more precision and effectiveness to create plasmid DNA-based vaccines. These techniques significantly increase the possibilities of creating DNA vaccines that are synthetic by enabling the seamless assembly of many DNA fragments, as well as precise editing of genetic sequences in turn (Ashique et al., 2023a; Choi & Berdis, 2019).

3.1.2 Vector optimization

With the news of DNA vaccines, great attention has been paid to vector optimization since the performance of the vaccine depends highly on the efficacy of expression and delivery. The feasibility and robustness of plasmid vectors that can be employed in DNA vaccinogens are to be secured to achieve a high level of expression of antigens. That is why the selection of a promoter is an important factor when it comes to fine-tuning vectors. Initiating the transcription of the antigen-coding gene is the promoter; an essential DNA fragment. DNA vaccines can include strong active promoters and since the DNA is not integrated into the cells genome, it uses constitutive promoters such as CMV promoter that can greatly spur gene expression in numerous types of cells in the host (Suschak et al., 2017). Also, enhancers can increase transcriptional activity even more and increase overall efficacy (Paston et al., 2021). Thus, the incorporation of the regulatory elements that increase the stability of the mRNA as well as the efficiency of the translation is one of the crucial factors when designing the vectors. The structural elements consist of introns, polyadenylation sites and 5 3′ end of the mRNA molecule in addition to 5′UTR region. The stability of mRNA as well as efficacy of translation from OUTFs that may be optimized can lead to an increase in synthesis of antigens (Amanpour, 2021). In the code sequence introns can positively regulate genes through the export of nuclear RNA and through splicing (Villarreal et al., 2013).

Additionally, it's normal to integrate the antibiotic resistance indicators as well as the source of replication in bacterial plasmid vectors. These characteristics aid in the development and selection of bacteria that produce the plasmid throughout manufacturing (Wang et al., 2018).

Simple antimicrobial vectors have seen rapid development in vector optimization that reduces the chance of developing resistance to antibiotics and increases the safety profile of the vaccine overall. In addition, the efficacy and effectiveness of DNA vaccines are further improved with the advent of new methods of delivery, such as electroporation which boosts the rate of plasmid DNA transfer into the host cell (Vishweshwaraiah and Dokholyan, 2022; Oude Blenke et al., 2023).

3.2 Clinical trials: a historical overview

The promising clinical trials are being followed by constant progression from the beginning of research and preclinical studies in the past of the DNA and mRNA vaccines to treat cancer. In the beginning, this is now possible thanks to advancements in molecular biology the field of immunology, as well as delivery technologies that allowed these groundbreaking vaccines to become integral components of the cancer treatment strategies.

3.2.1 Key trials and results

Many important studies that have drastically improved our knowledge of the technology during DNA vaccines from their conception until their clinical use. In the case of HIV is one of the first clinical trials for trials of a DNA vaccine was completed during the 1990s. While this study proved that DNA vaccines aren't harmful but also demonstrated that it's difficult to complete substantial immunogenicity (Cui, 2005). Studies conducted in the following years have continued looking into the possibility of DNA vaccines in the treatment of a wide range of ailments, like infections and cancer. A notable example can be found in of the Trimble et al. (2015) study, which assessed the efficacy of the DNA vaccine targeted against human HPV (HPV) for women who had high-grade cervical lesions. The positive outcome of this study included an abundance of patients who showed lessening of lesions and strong immune responses to HPV Antigens similar to INO-3112, which is which is a DNA vaccine targeting cervical and head malignancies that are related to HPV as well, has shown notable immune response in the clinical trial that set the stage for further studies in DNA vaccines to fight cancer (Kim et al., 2014).

The COVID-19 has also created vaccines known as the DNA vaccines. INO-4800 was one of the DNA vaccine candidates developed by the

Inovio Pharmaceuticals and it got progressed rapidly in the phase of clinical trials. The experience of the first phase of trials showed that the vaccine was able to stimulate rather sound T-cell and antibody responses and was compatible, thus pointing at the advantages of DNA vaccine regarding the emergence of the new infectious diseases (Porter & Raviprakash, 2017).

Cichutek et al. conducted a significant study that concentrated on the development of a DNA vaccine for fighting the Ebola virus. The study provided the basis for the vaccine's use in outbreak situations by demonstrating its safety as well as the ability to trigger robust immune responses within the population (Sheets et al., 2006). The outcome of these studies highlights the flexibility and effectiveness of DNA vaccines for various medical fields.

3.2.2 Impact on vaccine development

The world of vaccine development has significantly been impacted by DNA vaccine clinical studies. The validation of the safety characteristics of DNA vaccines has been among of the most significant advancements. The payoff has increased confidence in their use and has prompted further investigation into their effectiveness for use in preventive and therapeutic settings (Lopes et al., 2019; Singh et al., 2024; Dwivedi et al., 2024).

The studies have also drawn attention to the need to develop better strategies for delivering vaccinations. The initial studies showed that powerful immune responses could not be achieved through standard injections into the intramuscular area. Therefore, innovative techniques for delivery such as electroporation which boosts the uptake of DNA by the cells and enhances immunogenicity were developed and later implemented (Wang & Yuan, 2024). Since then, electroporation is used as a standard method for giving DNA vaccines, significantly increasing the effectiveness of these vaccines. Additionally, an important outcome from research studies has been the capability of DNA vaccines to trigger cellular as well as humoral immune reactions. Particularly in the case of ongoing infections or cancers in which a powerful immune system is required to eliminate malignant or infected cells, this double reaction is crucial for the long-term success of the immune system (Xu et al., 2016).

Another major benefit of DNA vaccines is their ability to adapt quickly. The nature of these vaccines is synthetic, which allows for rapid production and modification to respond to emerging ailments. DNA-based vaccine contestants are among those very first to be tested in clinical trials during the COVID-19 epidemic, which demonstrated the potential of this vaccine to be deployed quickly during emergencies (Villarreal et al., 2013; Alamri et al., 2021).

In the end, the information gathered through clinical studies has led to improvements in vaccination development as well as administration and usage, which has established DNA vaccines as a useful and adaptable weapon for fighting many diseases (Dhoundiyal et al., 2024).

3.3 Overcoming challenges

3.3.1 Delivery mechanisms

Transfer of plasmid DNA to cells of the host is among the most difficult obstacles to the design of DNA-based vaccines. The antigen encoded must be successfully introduced into host cells for transcription and translation to occur and generate a powerful immune reaction. There are a variety of delivery strategies that are being investigated to increase DNA vaccination. The most studied way to improve DNA vaccine distribution is electroporation. By together short electrical pulses electroporation creates a hole in the cell membrane that allows for a more efficient introduction of the DNA plasmid. Electroporation has been proven to be effective and could significantly rise DNA vaccine efficacy and the effectiveness of transfection (Lu et al., 2024). Clinical trials have shown such as the transmission of a DNA vaccine to fight the human virus (HPV) together with electroporation produced an enhanced immune response specific to the antigen (Kichaev et al., 2013).

Using injectables that do not require needles such as jet injectors for quick injection of DNA vaccine directly into the skin or muscle is a different approach. With the removal of the need for needles, this method not only improves patients' compliance but also enhances the distribution of the vaccine within tissues, leading to improved absorbency of the cells (Ledesma-Feliciano et al., 2023). In the animal model, research has shown that giving an antigen-specific DNA vaccine to fight the influenza virus without needles produced strong immunity to cellular and humoral factors (Mooij et al., 2019).

The possibilities of with delivery techniques made of nanoparticles to boost the efficiency of DNA vaccines are also being investigated. These methods encapsulate DNA molecules in nanoparticles composed of polymers, lipids, or any other material, that stop degradation and increase the cellular process of intake. Nanoparticles that are self-adjuvant are effective in enhancing DNA vaccination efficacy by providing better antigen exposure for immune cells. Nanomaterials that deliver the vaccine have adjuvant properties (Shen et al., 2024).

Biodegradable polymers to construct nanoparticles for the DNA vaccines have been developed through use of polylactic-co-glycolic acid (PLGA). One can consider producing nanoparticles that enable DNA release with time lengthened immunity stimulation and antigens manifests. Thus, the immunization study utilizing the DNA based vaccines encapsulating in the PLGA nanoparticles had shown enhancements in the immunocompetent reaction and protection against tough pathogens (Bolhassani et al., 2014).

3.3.2 Immunogenicity and efficacy

DNA vaccines have been at least promising; however, clinical trials have revealed that immunogenicity with DNA vaccines is generally lower than anticipated. This implies that DNA vaccines have to increase the immune response that they elicit in order to be useful in treatment and prevention. Several measures have been used in an attempt to solve this problem. One way of increasing the efficiency of immunogenicity is through the addition of molecular adjuvants. It shall be noted that the adjuvants may be incorporated in conjunction with DNA vaccination in order to enhance the response to immunological stimuli. Till date, there are hundreds of cytokines, some of which include Interleukin-12 (IL-12) and Granulocyte Macrophage Colony Stimulating Factor (GM- CSF) which have been used to promote immune response by stimulating activation and proliferation of immune cells (Ashique et al., 2022). Several investigations have revealed that the increase in immune responses both the cell mediated and the humoral mediated by the administration of DNA vaccines and also adjuvants containing cytokines (Olsen, 2000; Farzanehpour et al., 2013).

Codon optimization is another method which helps in enhancement of the production of a DNA vaccine's antigen encoded in the DNA. It is done in such a manner that the DNA sequence is made to include codons that the host cellular machine can deal with in the best way possible hence producing more protein. Studies in the preclinical stage have shown an improvement in the immunogenicity of codon-optimized DNA vaccinations (Ko et al., 2005). Additionally, the efficacy of DNA vaccines is affected by the method of administration. Intradermal administration utilizes the extensive skin system of antigen-presenting cells (APCs) that include dendritic cells and is adept at presenting the antigen with greater effectiveness. Studies have demonstrated that, in comparison to intramuscular treatments, intradermal injection of DNA vaccines triggers higher immune reactions (Patel et al., 2021).

Employing heterologous prime booster strategies in which the DNA vaccine is used as a priming vaccine and another vaccine method that is a vector of virus or protein-based vaccination, functions as the booster – is another innovative method. Utilizing the benefits of multiple vaccination systems the strategy can increase the immunity response in general. Through clinical studies like this, for instance, an initial boost regimen that included an RNA vaccine and the use of virus-based vaccine vectors showed enhanced protection and immunogenicity to HIV (Sapkota et al., 2022; Peng et al., 2021).

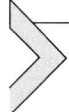

4. Advances in mRNA vaccine technology

4.1 mRNA synthesis and delivery

4.1.1 Lipid nanoparticle encapsulation

The lipid nanoparticle (LNP) encapsulation process is one of the biggest technological advances in the field of mRNA-based vaccines. The efficient dispersal of mRNA-based vaccines, particularly those designed for COVID-19 as the Pfizer-BioNTech or Moderna vaccines, has significantly improved by this technique. Lipids which make up LNPs are spherical which encloses DNA molecules in them and prevents their integrity from degrading (Lee et al., 2023).

For the creation of nanoparticles, MRNA is combined with lipids in carefully controlled conditions during the encapsulation process. The LNPs benefit the mRNA to enter cells much more quickly and also shield it from body nucleases. mRNA is then transported into the cytoplasm of cells and is transformed into the antigen of the target protein after the LNPs are joined to the membrane of cells (Xu et al., 2020; Kiaie et al., 2022).

The goal purpose of LNPs can be to boost the stability of mRNA as well as the effectiveness of its delivery. Most of them contain ionizable lipids that boost mRNA's endosomal escape and ensure that the majority of the mRNA released enters the cytoplasm intact. This process is vital in triggering an effective immune response (Yousefi Adlsadabad et al., 2024). Furthermore, by changing the surface properties of LNPs, LNPs can be made specifically targeted at specific tissues or cells, increasing the specificity of immune responses (Li et al., 2024).

LNPs greatly enhance the biodistribution of pharmacokinetics and distribution the mRNA-based vaccines. Studies have shown that vaccines made with mRNA encoded in LNPs produce lasting and robust immunological reactions which are evidenced by the increased level of T-cell reactions and neutralizing antibody (Ashique et al., 2023b). Compared to adjuvants that are This method has proven to have an excellent safety profile in clinical trials and has shown minimal adverse consequences (Shepherd et al., 2023).

Furthermore, the rapid development and production on a large scale of mRNA-based vaccines was achieved through the capacity of LNP production. Large-scale and consistent production of mRNA encapsulated by LNP, which is essential to satisfy the growing demand for vaccines across the globe is made possible through techniques such as the microfluidic mix (Ni, 2023).

4.1.2 Alternative delivery systems

Lipid nanoparticles were the principal ingredient in mRNA vaccine delivery, alternative delivery strategies are being studied to work past certain challenges and improve the effectiveness of mRNA vaccines. Utilizing nanoparticles made of polymers could be a choice. The capacity of polymers like polyethyleneimine (PEI) and poly(lactic-co-glycolic acid) (PLGA) to encapsulate and distribute mRNA has been studied (Witten et al., 2024). Polymers can form stable and robust structures with mRNA, protecting it from degrading and aiding in the absorption of mRNA by cells. The advantage of polymer-based delivery systems is their customizable properties, which permit an improvement in immunogenicity and distribution through changing the size of particles, their charge, and well surface attributes. It has been established that PEI improves the efficacy of transfection with mRNA, which results in higher levels of protein produced in the targeted cells (Bolhassani et al., 2014). But, PLGA offers a biodegradable matrix with the capability to allow the release of mRNA for longer periods of duration, which can raise the length of the response of the immune system (Bose et al., 2019).

A different interesting opportunity for the delivery of mRNA is nanoemulsions. They encapsulate mRNA making it easier to distribute and providing security together oils-in-water-based Emulsions. Increased stability of mRNA and its uptake from antigen-presenting cells (APCs) can be achieved using nanoemulsions. APCs are crucial for the triggering of the immune system (Huang et al., 2022). The research has demonstrated that nanoemulsions of mRNA have excellent safety profiles and may trigger a powerful immune response (Brazzoli et al., 2016). Encapsulation involves mixing mRNA and lipids in controlled conditions for the formation of nanoparticles.

Furthermore, to improve the efficacy of vaccines containing mRNA the use of cell-based delivery techniques is being studied. This includes delivering MRNA directly into the immune system through cells such as dendritic cells (DCs). Once the patient is given DCs, DCs that have been equipped with mRNA could be transferred to lymphoid organs, and deliver the antigen encoded for T cell delivery (Van Lint et al., 2014; Parums, 2021). This strategy leverages the natural capacity of DCs to stimulate and increase immune responses. This could lead to more efficient methods of vaccination.

4.2 Case studies: mRNA vaccines against cancer

4.2.1 Clinical applications

Studies on mRNA-based vaccines' possibilities for use in treating cancer have increased dramatically because of their efficacy in the COVID-19 outbreak. Cancer mRNA vaccines work by coding antigens specific to cancerous tumors. The body transforms into proteins to trigger the immune system's response against cancerous cells. This innovative method makes use of the body's resources to create the antigens at the targeted site and triggers an intense and specific immune reaction (Ankrah et al., 2023).

The clinical development of individualized neoantigen vaccinations is well-known as an example of using MRNA vaccines for cancer treatment. Specific changes that occur in a person's cancerous tissue, impart the basis for creating these vaccinations. Companies like BioNTech as well as Moderna have demonstrated the efficacy and efficacy of these customized MRNA vaccines through clinical tests (Shemesh et al., 2021; Wang et al., 2023b).

Using mRNA vaccinations with other immunotherapies offers an effective therapeutic option. Combining the mRNA vaccination CV9202 is a powerful vaccine that targets many antigens found in non-small-cell lung cancer (NSCLC) as well as checkpoint inhibitors has been proven to increase the outcomes of patients and increase the immunity system overall. Monotherapy's drawbacks can be overcome with this combination therapy offering a more complete regimen for treatments (Brazzoli et al., 2016).

Additionally, studies have been conducted on mRNA-based vaccines which target PSMA which is also known as prostate-specific membrane antigen for prostate cancer. The immunogenicity and safety of the Moderna mRNA-4157 vaccination have been evaluated through clinical studies. Initial findings indicate that the vaccine is highly stimulating to the immune system and is well tolerated, which opens the way for more tests to determine its effectiveness (Rosa et al., 2021; Chen et al., 2022).

4.2.2 Lessons from COVID-19 mRNA vaccine success

A wealth of important information that could be utilized in the design of cancer-specific vaccines have been gained from the rapid development and wide use of mRNA vaccines throughout the COVID-19 epidemic. Being able to develop, manufacture, and disseminate mRNA-based vaccines is crucial to the global reaction to COVID-19. It also shows that cancer vaccines can be rapidly developed in response to new needs (Morris & Kopetz, 2022).

In addition, highlights the importance of the importance of lipid nanoparticle (LNP) delivery technologies including COVID-19 vaccines. They have been proven extremely effective at stopping the mRNA from being destroyed and making it much easier to penetrate cells. Its ability to generate powerful immune responses together LNP-encapsulated MRNA vaccines has raised the potential of with the same delivery method for cancer-specific vaccines too. This has inspired more studies to determine the excellent methods to make LNPs to treat cancer (Shulman et al., 2022).

The value of large-scale clinical studies as well as real-world data to determine the efficacy and safety of vaccines is another vital knowledge. The vast data regarding the effectiveness of COVID-19 mRNA-based vaccines across different groups which can be attributed to the wide use of COVID-19 mRNA vaccines could benefit in the development and evaluation of the effectiveness and safety of these vaccines. In particular, the ability to monitor side effects as well as immune responses within a large group has helped in improving the formulation of vaccines as well as dosage regimens (Barbier et al., 2022).

Additionally, the collaboration between pharmaceutical companies as well as regulatory agencies and public health officials throughout the epidemic set an established standard for future study of vaccines. Working together and collaborating, we could speed up the process of approving cancer vaccines and ensure that those most likely participants are available to patients earlier. The fast-tracked regulatory processes for COVID-19 vaccines may be used as a reference to speed up approvals for cancer vaccines and still maintain the safety and effectiveness (Ashique et al., 2021).

The confidence of people in mRNA technology has grown because of the efficiency of COVID-19's mRNA vaccines. This can be crucial to the success of new cancer vaccines. Once cancer vaccines are readily available, awareness of their benefits and security will encourage them to use which will allow more patients access to the most cutting-edge treatments (Ladak et al., 2022).

In the end, the COVID-19 epidemic has provided us with invaluable lessons that can benefit to further develop the application of mRNA vaccines to aid in the fight against cancer. The development and use of mRNA-based cancer vaccines is possible by taking advantage of the speedy development of effective delivery techniques as well as the extensive trial data and the cooperative efforts that were demonstrated during the outbreak (Gupta et al., 2022).

4.3 Safety and regulatory aspects

4.3.1 Side effects and mitigation

The development and usage of mRNA vaccinations have been concentrated on the safety of their products. When the COVID-19 epidemic, mRNA vaccinations were used extensively, which resulted in a variety of data on their safety as well as adverse reactions. The outcome have shown that mRNA-based vaccines are very well-tolerated, with most side reactions being moderate to mild as well as temporary in their the nature of. There are local reactions at the injection location, including swelling, redness, or swelling, along with general reactions like anxiety, headache, fever as well as nausea, chills and fever is a common occurrence of mRNA vaccinations. The side effects typically disappear within a couple of days, and indicate the body's reaction to the vaccination in a way that is immunologically (Trimble et al., 2015; Sheets et al., 2006; Lin et al., 2015). Pericarditis and myocarditis are described as rare, but severe negative effects, particularly in older men following the second dose of the mRNA. COVID-19 vaccination (Liu et al., 2022).

Efforts have also been made to reduce the adverse effects of the policy measures that have been taken in relation to health care sector. This screening is important before administering the vaccine since it will help in identifying those individuals, body or immune system, which is likely to react badly to it. When vaccinations are given to all people Post-vaccination surveillance systems, which includes Vaccine Adverse Event Reporting System (VAERS) in the US becomes important in identifying and evaluating the safety of vaccines (Cheng et al., 2023; Ferner et al., 2022). These systems enable the identification of every prospective threat for safety and enable the regulators to respond swiftly. In addition to adjuvants, the delivery methods are a must when it comes to enhancing the immunogenicity and at the same time minimizing the side effects. In the case of currently used mRNA based vaccines, the LNPs have been finetuned in order to enhance the distribution capacity of these particles and to reduce their reactogenicity. The works for additional modifications of the new-generation LNPs and other methods which can enhance the safety of the mRNA vaccines are being carried out (Lee et al., 2023). In addition, the public's faith in vaccines is largely based upon open disclosure of potential adverse reactions and ways to deal with these. In order to reduce fears and boost vaccine acceptance can be achieved through clear guidelines about what you should expect after an injection and the perfect way to deal with the frequent adverse reactions (Mir and Mir, 2024).

4.3.2 Approval processes

In particular, especially during the COVID-19 outbreak, the regulation procedure for licensing mRNA vaccines has seen significant modifications. In the past, making and approving an mRNA vaccine involves several of rigorous preclinical and clinical trials to test the vaccine's safety, effectiveness as well as its efficacy. They are examined by regulators. The chapter could take several years. process. To speed up the distribution of COVID-19 vaccines regulators such as that of the World Health Organisation (WHO) as well as The European Medicines Agency (EMA) and the U.S. Food and Drug Administration (FDA) established quick approval routes throughout the outbreak. The routes comprised Conditional Marketing Authorizations (CMAs) as well as emergency Use Authorizations (EUAs), that allowed the vaccination and distribution of vaccines, while additional data were being sought (Trimble et al., 2015; Xu et al., 2016; Graña et al., 2022). Pharmacovigilance programs are utilized to evaluate the effectiveness of mRNA-based vaccines once they've been accepted for approval. The regulatory bodies require that vaccine manufacturers conduct post-marketing studies of surveillance as well as prepare periodic safety updates (Wolff-Holz & Weise, 2020).

The efficiency of the COVID-19 mRNA-based vaccines has highlighted that it is possible to use similar pathways for accelerated regulation of other urgent public health problems like cancer. To speed up the process of approval for mRNA-based vaccines against cancer as well as other ailments and to ensure that patients get treatment options more quickly in a manner that is consistent with rigorous safety and efficacy standards and regulatory frameworks that were developed during the epidemic can be utilized to create templates (Przybylowski et al., 2007; Dolgin, 2021). The speedy development and approval of mRNA-based vaccines have significantly benefited by the cooperation between government institutions, pharmaceutical firms as well as research organizations. The cooperative approach allows for an easier exchange of data and resources data and has expedited the process of regulating and increased the effectiveness of overall the research into vaccines (Barbier et al., 2022; Yao et al., 2024).

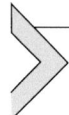

5. Clinical applications and efficacy

5.1 Evaluating clinical trials

5.1.1 Trial design and biomarker selection

A crucial aspect when assessing the efficacy and safety of mRNA as well as DNA vaccines is the design of clinical tests. The vaccines typically go through several phases of clinical trials. Probably the biggest component of design for trials is the choice of the biomarkers to be used in the trial. Some of the parameters that can be used as biomarkers include the amount of a specific substance found in body tissues or fluids or the changes patients undergo after receiving the therapy. As for DNA and mRNA vaccines, biomarkers may be specific immunological responses, such as the production of antibodies or stimulating the T-cells, and clinical outcomes, including the tumor's regression or the life completely free of disease (Suekane et al., 2020). Therefore, biomarkers can also identify the set of patients that is most likely to benefit from the treatment and also allow for a more accurate measurement of the effectiveness of vaccination. For instance, neoantigen-specific T-cell activity was chosen as the major read-out-marker for the phase 2 clinical trial of the mRNA vaccine for pancreatic cancer. The rationale for this decision was that it was considered that the vaccination might evoke a specific immune response to antigens that are selective to tumor cells. The study also showed the importance of the choice of biomarkers in the process of trials by focusing on the fact that people with robust T-cell responses recorded better results in the clinical trial (Singhai et al., 2024). The choice of the right biomarker is pivotal to adaptive trials, under which trial procedures are subject to change depending on the results of some finite tests. Besides, by allowing the discovery of efficacious treatments as well as eliminating ones that do not work, this system will increase the efficiency of clinical trials (Gergen & Petsch, 2022). Adaptive designs have been proven useful for the mRNA vaccine study where the classifying of patients and dosages were based on previously observed biomarkers (Wang et al., 2023b).

5.1.2 Data analysis and interpretation

Thus, in evaluation and analysis of the clinical trials data DNA and mRNA vaccine safety and efficacy scientifically correlates with the application of progress advanced statistical methods. Level of immunity as defined by T-cells together with antibody levels alongside clinical parameters such as ordinary survival, progression free survival and response rates are the most common endpoints of these clinical trials. One needs to understand the immune system that exists to provide an immune response after vaccinating, for data analysis to be possible. To assess the effectiveness of vaccination, it is necessary to make an extensive analysis of the correlation in the immunological system biomarkers and clinical results. Again, due to the potential confounding factors the application of the statistical models to establish the relationship between the levels of biomarkers and the outcome of the clinical trials (Vijayasingham et al., 2021; Liu et al., 2020). he evaluation of unfavorable events is another constituent of the analysis formula. In order to understand possible risks related to the vaccination process the security data require great attention and careful collection and analysis. It is important to keep watch for frequently occurring but potentially dangerous adverse reactions including reactions at the injection site and other general symptoms (Shulman et al., 2022).

Large data collections can be made more easily understood by using sophisticated data visualization tools, such as dashboards for monitoring immune function. Utilizing these tools, scientists can examine immune responses in time as well as across various groups of patients. This provides information on the mechanisms behind actions and possible predictors of responses (Liu et al., 2020; Metz et al., 2021).

5.2 Success stories in mRNA and DNA vaccines

5.2.1 Cancer-specific vaccine trials

DNA and mRNA vaccines, offering renewed hope of tailor-made chemotherapy for cancer. Customized MRNA vaccines targeting cancerous neoantigens among patients suffering from melanoma are a notable success story. Participants of a Phase I clinical trial received the customized mRNA vaccine which was developed with the mutations specific to them within their tumors. A few patients experienced a reduction in tumors following vaccination, which suggests the ability of mRNA vaccinations to create substantial anti-tumor immune responses (Fritsch & Ott, 2024).

In a Phase, IIb clinical trial of the VGX-3100 DNA vaccination a targeted HPV-16 and HPV-18, demonstrated remarkable efficacy for women suffering from CIN2 that is high-grade. (CIN2/3). DNA vaccines are able to aid in the prevention and treatment of cancer, as shown by the vaccination's strong immune response and Histological resection of lesions (Wu et al., 2011).

The application of mRNA vaccinations together with checkpoint inhibitors in the treatment of cancerous solid tumors is another instance of their effectiveness. For patients suffering from advanced melanoma, research that compared pembrolizumab, a PD-1 antibody, to an mRNA-based vaccine that encodes antigens associated with tumors showed better clinical outcomes as well as heightened immunity in comparison with pembrolizumab on its own (Van Lint et al., 2014; Ashique et al., 2024; Payandeh et al., 2019).

5.2.2 Immune response and patient outcomes

The efficacy of therapeutic DNA and mRNA vaccines are heavily dependent on the immune response they generate. The vaccines serve total protection from cancer through increasing the immune system's cellular and branching out into humoral structures. A case in point is the strong stimulation of CD4+ T-cells and CD8+cytotoxic T lymphocytes have been observed as part of the immunological response to mRNA vaccinations found in clinical tests. This is essential to eliminating cancerous cells and halting the recurrence of cancer. In addition, it's been established that mRNA vaccinations generate long-lasting memories that prepare long-term prevention of cancer (Shroff et al., 2021).

Results from clinical trials have been positive and several patients have shown noticeable improvements in their clinical condition. Patients participating in a clinical trial with an mRNA-based vaccine against colorectal cancer showed longer total and non-progression-free survival indicating the possibility of the vaccines improve longer-term outcome (Au et al., 2021; Indar et al., 2002).

Additionally, more targeted treatments that have fewer negative side effects, as well as greater effectiveness, can be attributed to the personalized nature of mRNA and DNA vaccines compatible with the patient's profile. The high specificity of identifying cancer cells and preserving healthy tissue can be demonstrated with personalized vaccinations that improve the safety of patients and their health (Shemesh et al., 2021; Fritsch & Ott, 2024).

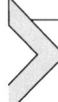

6. Challenges and opportunities
6.1 Scale-up and mass production

6.1.1 Technological and logistic barriers

The production of DNA and mRNA-based vaccines needs to be scaled up in order to meet the global demand which will mean overcoming significant technological and logistical obstacles. Manufacturing is among the biggest technological challenges. In particular, the production of vaccines containing mRNA requires sophisticated equipment that can handle the process of

RNA synthesis, purification, and formulation issues. Making sure that the integrity and stability of mRNA is a vital element in this procedure because it is extremely susceptible to degrading (Abu Esba et al., 2020).

Many obstacles to the production of Lipid nanoparticles (LNPs) are necessary for the delivery of vaccine mRNA. To encapsulate MRNA, protect it from destruction, and allow it to penetrate the human cell, the nanoparticles need to be crafted with great care. strict quality control protocols and the most cutting-edge technologies are essential to warrant that LNP production grows to warrant uniformity and efficiency (Shepherd et al., 2023).The distribution of DNA and mRNA vaccines can pose logistical difficulties. In order to maintain their stability, the vaccines are often required to be shipped and kept within the form of a cold chain. Certain mRNA-based vaccines are a good example. They must be stored at very low temperatures. Although this can be done in countries with high incomes, however, it is a major issue in the low and middle-income regions because these locations lack the infrastructure for cold storage (Rosa et al., 2021). The cost and difficulty of distribution are increased due to the necessity for freezers that are specialized and have continuous temperature control. Additionally, during times of huge demand the supply chain of the raw materials, such as lipids enzymes, and nucleotides needed to make vaccines can become overwhelmed. The production or distribution of vaccinations can be delayed because of supply chain interruptions. Making investments in the development of manufacturing abilities and coordination of international efforts are essential in order to assure the availability of this vital mineral (Buck et al., 2024).

6.1.2 Economic considerations

There are many financial factors to be considered when expanding the production of vaccines. Production facilities, machines, and other technology are accompanied by the expense of a large upfront investment. Private and public companies should set aside a substantial sum to establish and improve production facilities so that are able to meet the demands of global vaccination programmes (Barbier et al., 2022).

Additionally, it's expensive to maintain cold chain logistics of mRNA vaccinations. This covers the cost of temperature-controlled shipping, specialized storage containers, and monitoring systems to guarantee the vaccinations stay effective until they are administered to the final recipients. The costs can be prohibitive, especially for countries in need that require International financial aid and subsidy (Lu et al., 2024).

The cost of vaccinations is an extra aspect of economics. For universal vaccination, vaccines need to be affordable, however, they must take into account the costs that are associated with development manufacturing, production, and distribution. Innovative financial strategies, such as tied pricing, partnerships between public and private as well and international financing programs like COVAX will be required in order to attain a balance between the sustainability of affordability (Shulman et al., 2022; Ferner et al., 2022; Abu Esba et al., 2020).

Effective immunization strategies could have a significant impact on the economy. Through preventing illnesses, decreasing the necessity for hospitalization as well as facilitating faster return to work In the end, effective vaccinations will reduce costs for healthcare. It is therefore feasible to consider the investment in infrastructure for vaccines and production capacities as a plan of finance that is beneficial to both economic and public health security (Rahman et al., 2021b).

6.2 Future research directions

6.2.1 Combining therapies

An intriguing method to boost the efficacy and extend the usage of mRNA, as well as DNA vaccines, is to mix these with other treatments. Combining vaccines and immune checkpoint inhibitors is one of these strategies. Checkpoint inhibitors, such as CTLA-4 and PD-1-1/PD-L1 inhibitors work by blocking the protein which stops T-cells in their fight against cancer cells. This strengthens your immune system. The research has shown that a combination of checkpoint inhibitors and cancer vaccines may boost the immune system against tumors and result in improved outcomes for patients (Ashique et al., 2024; Payandeh et al., 2019).

Oncolytic virus-based vaccines are a more exciting mix. Oncolytic viruses trigger an immune reaction that is tumor-defying with the intention of specifically eliminating cancerous cells. They can display tumor Antigens much more efficaciously and enhance the immune system if combined with DNA or mRNA vaccines that could raise the effectiveness of treatments for cancer (Le et al., 2022).

Additionally, there could be advantages in combining vaccinations and traditional treatments such as chemotherapy or radiation. They can trigger the death of immune cells, which release antigens from tumors that your immune system could attack. Vaccines could enhance the reaction by providing extra antigens, as well as increasing the overall levels of activated immune cells (Verbeke et al., 2022; Santoro et al., 2018; Meng et al., 2019).

6.2.2 Next-generation vaccine platforms

The next-generation vaccination platforms aim to increase the efficacy of vaccines, their safety, and accessibility by addressing the limitations of current technologies. Self-amplifying RNA (siRNA) vaccines can be described as just one specific area. SaRNA vaccines, as opposed to conventional mRNA-based vaccines, include both antigens and the necessary components needed to replicate RNA. This means that fewer doses are needed to trigger the same level of immune reaction, which could cut the cost of production and reduce availability limitations (Gupta et al., 2022).

The use of artificial nanoparticles that mimic viruses is a different exciting avenue. It's possible to make viruses-like particles (VLPs) which exhibit an array of antigens that stimulate powerful immune responses, with no risk of spreading the disease. It has been clinically demonstrated that other VLP-based vaccinations which are being researched for various kinds of cancers and viral illnesses are very useful (Yousefi Adlsadabad et al., 2024; Witten et al., 2024; Huang et al., 2022). There is, therefore, a need to continue with the development of personalized cancer vaccines. The vaccines are developed to be used in specific Neoantigens and are completely personalized to join the characteristics of every solitary tumor patient's genetics. The Discovery of neoantigens in such patients and the development of personal vaccines became possible owing to the great progress in the field of bioinformatics and genetic sequencing. Some of clinical studies have shown that such personalized approaches can produce robust and antigen-specific immunities and enhance the outcomes among patients (Fritsch & Ott, 2024). There is another interesting direction that concerns applying machine learning and artificial intelligence or AI in the formation of vaccines. AI might enhance the design of vaccines, and discover the best antigens in a shorter time than humans by predicting the reaction of a patient when vaccinated. This is the main strategy that will improve the accuracy in the formulation of vaccines and highly reduce the period for development (Wang et al., 2023a).

7. Conclusion

A major shift in the treatment of cancer through chemotherapy was the emergence of mRNA & DNA vaccines. These new vaccines utilize the body pool of genes in order to produce cancers specific antigens. They elicit high and selective forms of specific immunity and possess numerous possibilities of being utilized in cancer prophylaxis as well as treatment. Throughout this chapter, mechanisms through which the DNA and mRNA vaccines function have revealed some features that make them different from traditional vaccines. These vaccinations act as useful tool to mitigate the genetics and immune evading ability of cancer as they are effective, specific and have relatively shorter periods of development. From the existing clinical trials, much has been realized on the effectiveness of these vaccines due to positive payoff in various forms of cancer. The mRNA-specific vaccines are promising for treatment of cancers associated with HPV and melanoma among many other illnesses. These are very good sample of how they can be used to show how such technologies. The trials show how crucial biomarkers are in controlling vaccination development and enhancing treatment strategies. Despite all these advancements, there are still a number of issues. The logistical and technological obstacles are between large-scale production and the scaling up of DNA and mRNA-based vaccines. This is mostly due to logistics for cold chain and manufacturing processes. Factors that affect the economy, like the cost of distribution and production need creative financial strategies that will make sure the vaccine is accessible to everyone around the world. Research avenues in the future are likely to boost the efficiency and effectiveness of the DNA and mRNA vaccines. The synergy of treatments, such as immune checkpoint inhibitors as well as cancer-causing viruses might be feasible if these vaccines are integrated with other therapies. Additionally, the development of next-generation vaccine platforms like self-amplifying RNA and virus-like particles could outshine the current limitations and revolutionize chemotherapy for cancer. The development of DNA as well as mRNA vaccines, from laboratory to bedside is a testament to the effectiveness of cooperation between scientists as well as the power of creativity. DNA and mRNA-based vaccines will revolutionize the way we treat cancer, as we try to unravel the nature of cancer and boost the effectiveness of these innovative technologies which will help provide hope for better, more personalized effective treatments.

References

Abu Esba, L. C., Al-Abdulkarim, H. A., Alrushidan, A., & Al Harbi, M. (2020). Pharmacy and therapeutics committee preparedness plan for COVID-19. *Global Journal on Quality and Safety in Healthcare, 3*(2), 55–64.

Alamri, S. S., Alluhaybi, K. A., Alhabbab, R. Y., Basabrain, M., Algaissi, A., Almahboub, S., et al. (2021). Synthetic SARS-CoV-2 spike-based DNA vaccine elicits robust and long-lasting Th1 humoral and cellular immunity in mice. *Frontiers in Microbiology, 12*, 727455.

Amanpour, S. (2021). The rapid development and early success of Covid 19 vaccines have raised hopes for accelerating the cancer treatment mechanism. *Archives of Razi Institute, 76*(1), 1–6.

Ankrah, P. K., Ilesanmi, A., Akinyemi, A. O., Lasehinde, V., Adurosakin, O. E., & Ajayi, O. H. (2023). Clinical analysis and applications of mRNA vaccines in infectious diseases and cancer treatment. *Cureus, 15*(10), e46354.

Ashique, S., Afzal, O., Hussain, A., Zeyaullah, M., Altamimi, M. A., Mishra, N., ... Anand, K. (2023a). It's all about plant derived natural phytoconstituents and phytonanomedicine to control skin cancer. *Journal of Drug Delivery Science and Technology, 84*, 104495.

Ashique, S., Almohaywi, B., Haider, N., Yasmin, S., Hussain, A., Mishra, N., & Garg, A. (2022). siRNA-based nanocarriers for targeted drug delivery to control breast cancer. *Advances in Cancer Biology-Metastasis, 4*, 100047.

Ashique, S., Bhowmick, M., Pal, R., Khatoon, H., Kumar, P., Sharma, H., ... Das, U. (2024). Multi drug resistance in colorectal cancer-approaches to overcome, advancements and future success. *Advances in Cancer Biology-Metastasis*, 100114.

Ashique, S., Hussain, A., Fatima, N., & Altamimi, M. A. (2023b). HPV pathogenesis, various types of vaccines, safety concern, prophylactic and therapeutic applications to control cervical cancer, and future perspective. *Virus Disease, 34*(2), 172–190.

Ashique, S., Sandhu, N. K., Chawla, V., & Chawla, P. A. (2021). Targeted drug delivery: Trends and perspectives. *Current Drug Delivery, 18*(10), 1435–1455.

Au, L., Fendler, A., Shepherd, S. T. C., Rzeniewicz, K., Cerrone, M., Byrne, F., et al. (2021). Cytokine release syndrome in a patient with colorectal cancer after vaccination with BNT162b2. *Nature Medicine, 27*(8), 1362–1366.

Barbier, A. J., Jiang, A. Y., Zhang, P., Wooster, R., & Anderson, D. G. (2022). The clinical progress of mRNA vaccines and immunotherapies. *Nature Biotechnology, 40*(6), 840–854.

Bolhassani, A., Javanzad, S., Saleh, T., Hashemi, M., Aghasadeghi, M. R., & Sadat, S. M. (2014). Polymeric nanoparticles: Potent vectors for vaccine delivery targeting cancer and infectious diseases. *Human Vaccines & Immunotherapeutics, 10*(2), 321–332.

Borzova, E. (2024). Global biotechnology leapfrogging during the COVID-19 pandemic: A trend to stay? *Trends in Biotechnology*, S0167-7799(24)00146-X.

Bose, R. J., Kim, M., Chang, J. H., Paulmurugan, R., Moon, J. J., Koh, W. G., et al. (2019). Biodegradable polymers for modern vaccine development. *Journal of Industrial and Engineering Chemistry Seoul Korea, 77*, 12–24.

Brazzoli, M., Magini, D., Bonci, A., Buccato, S., Giovani, C., Kratzer, R., et al. (2016). Induction of broad-based immunity and protective efficacy by self-amplifying mRNA vaccines encoding influenza virus hemagglutinin. *Journal of Virology, 90*(1), 332–344.

Buck, P. O., Gomes, D. A., Beck, E., Kirson, N., Mattera, M., Carroll, S., et al. (2024). New vaccine platforms-novel dimensions of economic and societal value and their measurement. *Vaccines, 12*(3), 234.

Chakraborty, S., & Rahman, T. (2012). The difficulties in cancer treatment. *Ecancermedicalscience, 6*, ed16.

Chaudhary, N., Weissman, D., & Whitehead, K. A. (2021). mRNA vaccines for infectious diseases: Principles, delivery and clinical translation. *Nature Reviews. Drug Discovery, 20*(11), 817–838.

Chen, J., Ye, Z., Huang, C., Qiu, M., Song, D., Li, Y., et al. (2022). Lipid nanoparticle-mediated lymph node-targeting delivery of mRNA cancer vaccine elicits robust CD8+ T cell response. *Proceedings of the National Academy of Sciences of the United States of America, 119*(34), e2207841119.

Cheng, F., Wang, Y., Bai, Y., Liang, Z., Mao, Q., Liu, D., et al. (2023). Research advances on the stability of mRNA vaccines. *Viruses, 15*(3), 668.

Choi, J. S., & Berdis, A. (2019). Artificial nucleosides as diagnostic probes to measure translesion DNA synthesis. *Methods in Molecular Biology (Clifton, N.J.), 1973*, 237–249.

Cui, Z. (2005). DNA vaccine. *Advances in Genetics, 54*, 257–289.

David, F., Davis, A. M., Gossing, M., Hayes, M. A., Romero, E., Scott, L. H., et al. (2021). A perspective on synthetic biology in drug discovery and development-current impact and future opportunities. *SLAS DISCOVERY: Advancing the Science of Drug, 26*(5), 581–603.

Debela, D. T., Muzazu, S. G., Heraro, K. D., Ndalama, M. T., Mesele, B. W., Haile, D. C., et al. (2021). New approaches and procedures for cancer treatment: Current perspectives. *SAGE Open Medicine, 9*, 20503121211034366.

Dede, Z., Tumer, K., Kan, T., & Yucel, B. (2023). Current advances and future prospects in cancer immunotherapeutics. *Medeniyet Medical Journal, 38*(1), 88–94.

Dhoundiyal, S., Srivastava, S., Kumar, S., Singh, G., Ashique, S., Pal, R., ... Taghizadeh-Hesary, F. (2024). Radiopharmaceuticals: navigating the frontier of precision medicine and therapeutic innovation. *European Journal of Medical Research, 29*(1), 26.

Dolgin, E. (2021). The tangled history of mRNA vaccines. *Nature, 597*(7876), 318–324.

Dwivedi, Singh, S., Agrawal, V., Misra, R., Sadashiv, R., Fatima, G., et al. (2024). Human monkeypox virus and host immunity: New challenges in diagnostics and treatment strategies. *Advances in Experimental Medicine and Biology, 1451*, 219–237.

Farzanehpour, M., Soleimanjahi, H., Hassan, Z. M., Amanzadeh, A., Ghaemi, A., & Fazeli, M. (2013). HSP70 modified response against HPV based tumor. *European Review for Medical and Pharmacological Sciences, 17*(2), 228–234.

Feeley, T. W., Sledge, G. W., Levit, L., & Ganz, P. A. (2014). Improving the quality of cancer care in America through health information technology. *Journal of the American Medical Informatics Association JAMIA, 21*(5), 772–775.

Ferner, R. E., Stevens, R. J., Anton, C., & Aronson, J. K. (2022). Spontaneous reporting to regulatory authorities of suspected adverse drug reactions to COVID-19 vaccines over time: The effect of publicity. *Drug Safety: An International Journal of Medical Toxicology and Drug Experience, 45*(2), 137–144.

Föhse, K., Geckin, B., Zoodsma, M., Kilic, G., Liu, Z., Röring, R. J., et al. (2023a). The impact of BNT162b2 mRNA vaccine on adaptive and innate immune responses. *Clinical Immunology (Orlando, Fla.), 255*, 109762.

Föhse, K., Geckin, B., Zoodsma, M., Kilic, G., Liu, Z., Röring, R. J., et al. (2023b). The impact of BNT162b2 mRNA vaccine on adaptive and innate immune responses. *Clinical Immunology (Orlando, Fla.), 255*, 109762.

Foulkes, I., & Sharpless, N. E. (2021). Cancer grand challenges: Embarking on a new era of discovery. *Cancer Discovery, 11*(1), 23–27.

Fritsch, E. F., & Ott, P. A. (2024). Personalized cancer vaccines directed against tumor mutations: Building evidence from mice to humans. *Cancer Research, 84*(7), 953–955.

Galmarini, C. M. (2020). Why we do what we do. A brief analysis of cancer therapies. *EXCLI Journal, 19*, 1401–1413.

Garg, A., Kaity, S., Thakur, M., Datusalia, A., & Kumar, A. (2023). *Future Prospective and Challenges in the Treatment of Cancer*, 382–394.

Gergen, J., & Petsch, B. (2022). mRNA-based vaccines and mode of action. *Current Topics in Microbiology and Immunology, 440*, 1–30.

Gomez, A. M., Babuadze, G. G., Plourde-Campagna, M. A., Azizi, H., Berger, A., Kozak, R., et al. (2022). A novel intradermal tattoo-based injection device enhances the immunogenicity of plasmid DNA vaccines. *NPJ Vaccines, 7*(1), 172.

Gote, V., Bolla, P. K., Kommineni, N., Butreddy, A., Nukala, P. K., Palakurthi, S. S., et al. (2023). A comprehensive review of mRNA vaccines. *International Journal of Molecular Sciences, 24*(3), 2700.

Graña, C., Ghosn, L., Evrenoglou, T., Jarde, A., Minozzi, S., Bergman, H., et al. (2022). Efficacy and safety of COVID-19 vaccines. *Cochrane Database of Systematic Reviews (Online), 12*(12), CD015477.

Gupta, M., Wahi, A., Sharma, P., Nagpal, R., Raina, N., Kaurav, M., et al. (2022). Recent Advances in Cancer Vaccines: Challenges, achievements, and futuristic prospects. *Vaccines, 10*(12), 2011.

Hani, U., Gowda, B. J., Haider, N., Ramesh, K. V., Paul, K., Ashique, S., ... Kesharwani, P. (2023). Nanoparticle-based approaches for treatment of hematological malignancies: A comprehensive review. *AAPS PharmSciTech, 24*(8), 233.

Heine, A., Juranek, S., & Brossart, P. (2021). Clinical and immunological effects of mRNA vaccines in malignant diseases. *Molecular Cancer, 20*(1), 52.

Huang, T., Peng, L., Han, Y., Wang, D., He, X., Wang, J., et al. (2022). Lipid nanoparticle-based mRNA vaccines in cancers: Current advances and future prospects. *Frontiers in Immunology, 13*, 922301.

Indar, A., Maxwell-Armstrong, C. A., Durrant, L. G., Carmichael, J., & Scholefield, J. H. (2002). Current concepts in immunotherapy for the treatment of colorectal cancer. *Journal of the Royal College of Surgeons of Edinburgh, 47*(2), 458–474.

Kiaie, S. H., Majidi Zolbanin, N., Ahmadi, A., Bagherifar, R., Valizadeh, H., Kashanchi, F., et al. (2022). Recent advances in mRNA-LNP therapeutics: Immunological and pharmacological aspects. *Journal of Nanobiotechnology, 20*(1), 276.

Kichaev, G., Mendoza, J. M., Amante, D., Smith, T. R. F., McCoy, J. R., Sardesai, N. Y., et al. (2013). Electroporation mediated DNA vaccination directly to a mucosal surface results in improved immune responses. *Human Vaccines & Immunotherapeutics, 9*(10), 2041–2048.

Kim, T. J., Jin, H. T., Hur, S. Y., Yang, H. G., Seo, Y. B., Hong, S. R., et al. (2014). Clearance of persistent HPV infection and cervical lesion by therapeutic DNA vaccine in CIN3 patients. *Nature Communications, 5*, 5317.

Ko, H. J., Ko, S. Y., Kim, Y. J., Lee, E. G., Cho, S. N., & Kang, C. Y. (2005). Optimization of codon usage enhances the immunogenicity of a DNA vaccine encoding mycobacterial antigen Ag85B. *Infection and Immunity, 73*(9), 5666–5674.

Kumar, A. R., Devan, A. R., Nair, B., Vinod, B. S., & Nath, L. R. (2021). Harnessing the immune system against cancer: Current immunotherapy approaches and therapeutic targets. *Molecular Biology Reports, 48*(12), 8075–8095.

Kutzler, M. A., & Weiner, D. B. (2008). DNA vaccines: Ready for prime time? *Nature Reviews. Genetics, 9*(10), 776–788.

Ladak, R. J., He, A. J., Huang, Y. H., & Ding, Y. (2022). The current landscape of mRNA vaccines against viruses and cancer—A mini review. *Frontiers in Immunology, 13*, 885371.

Le, I., Dhandayuthapani, S., Chacon, J., Eiring, A. M., & Gadad, S. S. (2022). Harnessing the immune system with cancer vaccines: From prevention to therapeutics. *Vaccines, 10*(5), 816.

Ledesma-Feliciano, C., Chapman, R., Hooper, J. W., Elma, K., Zehrung, D., Brennan, M. B., et al. (2023). Improved DNA vaccine delivery with needle-free injection systems. *Vaccines, 11*(2), 280.

Lee, Y., Jeong, M., Park, J., Jung, H., & Lee, H. (2023). Immunogenicity of lipid nanoparticles and its impact on the efficacy of mRNA vaccines and therapeutics. *Experimental & Molecular Medicine, 55*(10), 2085–2096.

Li, X., Qi, J., Wang, J., Hu, W., Zhou, W., Wang, Y., et al. (2024). Nanoparticle technology for mRNA: Delivery strategy, clinical application and developmental landscape. *Theranostics, 14*(2), 738–760.

Li, Y., Wang, M., Peng, X., Yang, Y., Chen, Q., Liu, J., et al. (2023). mRNA vaccine in cancer therapy: Current advance and future outlook. *Clinical and Translational Medicine, 13*(8), e1384.

Lin, M., Yuan, Y., Xu, J., Cai, X., Liu, S., Niu, L., et al. (2015). Safety and efficacy study of nasopharyngeal cancer stem cell vaccine. *Immunology Letters, 165*(1), 26–31.

Liu, B., Wang, Y. Z., Yin, X., Deng, X., Su, Y., Zhang, Y., et al. (2020). The consideration about safety data analysis and expression in instructions of vaccine clinic trials. *54*(3), 250–255.

Liu, M. A., Zhou, T., Sheets, R. L., Meyer, H., & Knezevic, I. (2022). WHO informal consultation on regulatory considerations for evaluation of the quality, safety and efficacy of RNA-based prophylactic vaccines for infectious diseases, 20-22 April 2021. *Emerging Microbes & Infections, 11*(1), 384–391.

Liu, M. A. (2019). A comparison of plasmid DNA and mRNA as vaccine technologies. *Vaccines, 7*(2), 37.

Lopes, A., Vandermeulen, G., & Préat, V. (2019). Cancer DNA vaccines: Current preclinical and clinical developments and future perspectives. *Journal of Experimental & Clinical Cancer Research CR, 38*(1), 146.

Lorentzen, C. L., Haanen, J. B., Met, Ö., & Svane, I. M. (2022). Clinical advances and ongoing trials on mRNA vaccines for cancer treatment. *The Lancet Oncology, 23*(10), e450–e458.

Lu, B., Lim, J. M., Yu, B., Song, S., Neeli, P., Sobhani, N., et al. (2024). The next-generation DNA vaccine platforms and delivery systems: Advances, challenges and prospects. *Frontiers in Immunology, 15*, 1332939.

Macheret, M., & Halazonetis, T. D. (2015). DNA replication stress as a hallmark of cancer. *Annual Review of Pathology, 10*, 425–448.

Matthews, H. K., Bertoli, C., & De Bruin, R. A. M. (2022). Cell cycle control in cancer. *Nature Reviews. Molecular Cell Biology, 23*(1), 74–88.

Meng, Z., Chen, Y., & Lu, M. (2019). Advances in targeting the innate and adaptive immune systems to cure chronic hepatitis B virus infection. *Frontiers in Immunology, 10*, 3127.

Metz, M., Smith, R., Mitchell, R., Duong, Y. T., Brown, K., Kinchen, S., et al. (2021). Data architecture to support real-time data analytics for the population-based HIV impact assessments. *Journal of Acquired Immune Deficiency Syndrome 1999, 87*(1), S28–S35.

Miao, L., Zhang, Y., & Huang, L. (2021). mRNA vaccine for cancer immunotherapy. *Molecular Cancer, 20*(1), 41.

Mir, S., & Mir, M. (2024). The mRNA vaccine, a swift warhead against a moving infectious disease target. *Expert Review of Vaccines, 23*(1), 336–348.

Mooij, P., Grødeland, G., Koopman, G., Andersen, T. K., Mortier, D., Nieuwenhuis, I. G., et al. (2019). Needle-free delivery of DNA: Targeting of hemagglutinin to MHC class II molecules protects rhesus macaques against H1N1 influenza. *Vaccine, 37*(6), 817–826.

Morris, V. K., & Kopetz, S. (2022). Don't blame the messenger: Lessons learned for cancer mRNA vaccines during the COVID-19 pandemic. *Nature Reviews. Cancer, 22*(6), 317–318.

Ni, L. (2023). Advances in mRNA-based cancer vaccines. *Vaccines, 11*(10), 1599.

Olsen, C. W. (2000). DNA vaccination against influenza viruses: A review with emphasis on equine and swine influenza. *Veterinary Microbiology, 74*(1–2), 149–164.

Oude Blenke, E., Örnskov, E., Schöneich, C., Nilsson, G. A., Volkin, D. B., Mastrobattista, E., et al. (2023). The storage and in-use stability of mRNA vaccines and therapeutics: Not a cold case. *Journal of Pharmaceutical Sciences, 112*(2), 386–403.

Pandya, A., Shah, Y., Kothari, N., Postwala, H., Shah, A., Parekh, P., et al. (2023). The future of cancer immunotherapy: DNA vaccines leading the way. *Medical Oncology (Northwood, London, England), 40*(7), 200.

Pardi, N., Hogan, M. J., Porter, F. W., & Weissman, D. (2018). mRNA vaccines - A new era in vaccinology. *Nature Reviews. Drug Discovery, 17*(4), 261–279.

Parums, D. V. (2021). Editorial: mRNA Vaccines and Immunotherapy in Oncology: A New Era for Personalized Medicine. *Medical Science Monitor: International Medical Journal for Experimental and Clinical Research, 27*, e933088.

Paston, S. J., Brentville, V. A., Symonds, P., & Durrant, L. G. (2021). Cancer vaccines, adjuvants, and delivery systems. *Frontiers in Immunology, 12*, 627932.

Patel, A., Reuschel, E. L., Xu, Z., Zaidi, F. I., Kim, K. Y., Scott, D. P., et al. (2021). Intradermal delivery of a synthetic DNA vaccine protects macaques from Middle East respiratory syndrome coronavirus. *JCI Insight, 6*(10), 146082, e146082.

Payandeh, Z., Yarahmadi, M., Nariman-Saleh-Fam, Z., Tarhriz, V., Islami, M., Aghdam, A. M., et al. (2019). Immune therapy of melanoma: Overview of therapeutic vaccines. *Journal of Cellular Physiology, 234*(9), 14612–14621.

Peng, S., Ferrall, L., Gaillard, S., Wang, C., Chi, W. Y., Huang, C. H., et al. (2021). Development of DNA vaccine targeting E6 and E7 proteins of human papillomavirus 16 (HPV16) and HPV18 for immunotherapy in combination with recombinant vaccinia boost and PD-1 antibody. *mBio, 12*(1), e03224-20.

Pilkington, E. H., Suys, E. J. A., Trevaskis, N. L., Wheatley, A. K., Zukancic, D., Algarni, A., et al. (2021). From influenza to COVID-19: Lipid nanoparticle mRNA vaccines at the frontiers of infectious diseases. *Acta Biomaterialia, 131*, 16–40.

Porter, K. R., & Raviprakash, K. (2017). DNA vaccine delivery and improved immunogenicity. *Current Issues in Molecular Biology, 22*, 129–138.

Przybylowski, M., Bartido, S., Borquez-Ojeda, O., Sadelain, M., & Rivière, I. (2007). Production of clinical-grade plasmid DNA for human Phase I clinical trials and large animal clinical studies. *Vaccine, 25*(27), 5013–5024.

Rahman, M. M., Zhou, N., & Huang, J. (2021a). An overview on the development of mRNA-based vaccines and their formulation strategies for improved antigen expression in vivo. *Vaccines, 9*(3), 244.

Rahman, S., Montero, M. T. V., Rowe, K., Kirton, R., & Kunik, F. (2021b). Epidemiology, pathogenesis, clinical presentations, diagnosis and treatment of COVID-19: A review of current evidence. *Expert Review of Clinical Pharmacology, 14*(5), 601–621.

Rosa, S. S., Prazeres, D. M. F., Azevedo, A. M., & Marques, M. P. C. (2021). mRNA vaccines manufacturing: Challenges and bottlenecks. *Vaccine, 39*(16), 2190–2200.

S, Venishaa, Kumar, P., Sen, A., Anand, A., Kaushik, M., Bhowmick M., et al. Unlocking the role of virus-like particles (VLPs) for cancer treatment. Curr Cancer Therapy Reviews, 20, 1–27. https://doi.org/10.2174/0115733947308351240514182503.

Sakib, M. N., Butt, Z. A., Morita, P. P., Oremus, M., Fong, G. T., & Hall, P. A. (2020). Considerations for an individual-level population notification system for pandemic response: A review and prototype. *Journal of Medical Internet Research, 22*(6), e19930.

Santoro, F., Pettini, E., Kazmin, D., Ciabattini, A., Fiorino, F., Gilfillan, G. D., et al. (2018). Transcriptomics of the vaccine immune response: Priming with adjuvant modulates recall innate responses after boosting. *Frontiers in Immunology, 9*, 1248.

Sapkota, B., Saud, B., Shrestha, R., Al-Fahad, D., Sah, R., Shrestha, S., et al. (2022). Heterologous prime-boost strategies for COVID-19 vaccines. *Journal of Travel Medicine: Official Publication of the International Society of Travel Medicine and the Asia Pacific Travel Health Association, 29*(3), taab191.

Sayour, E. J., Boczkowski, D., Mitchell, D. A., & Nair, S. K. (2024). Cancer mRNA vaccines: Clinical advances and future opportunities. *Nature Reviews Clinical Oncology*.

Schilsky, R. L., Allen, J., Benner, J., Sigal, E., & McClellan, M. (2010). Commentary: Tackling the challenges of developing targeted therapies for cancer. *The Oncologist, 15*(5), 484–487.

Sheets, R. L., Stein, J., Manetz, T. S., Andrews, C., Bailer, R., Rathmann, J., et al. (2006). Toxicological safety evaluation of DNA plasmid vaccines against HIV-1, Ebola, Severe Acute Respiratory Syndrome, or West Nile virus is similar despite differing plasmid backbones or gene-inserts. *Toxicological Sciences Official Journal of the Society of Toxicology, 91*(2), 620–630.

Shemesh, C. S., Hsu, J. C., Hosseini, I., Shen, B. Q., Rotte, A., Twomey, P., et al. (2021). Personalized cancer vaccines: Clinical landscape, challenges, and opportunities. *Molecular Therapy: The Journal of the American Society of Gene Therapy, 29*(2), 555–570.

Shen, F., Wang, H., Liu, Z., & Sun, L. (2024). DNA nanostructures: Self-adjuvant carriers for highly efficient subunit vaccines. *Angewandte Chemie (International Ed. in English), 63*(2), e202312624.

Shepherd, S. J., Han, X., Mukalel, A. J., El-Mayta, R., Thatte, A. S., Wu, J., et al. (2023). Throughput-scalable manufacturing of SARS-CoV-2 mRNA lipid nanoparticle vaccines. *Proceedings of the National Academy of Sciences of the United States of America, 120*(33), e2303567120.

Shroff, R. T., Chalasani, P., Wei, R., Pennington, D., Quirk, G., Schoenle, M. V., et al. (2021). Immune responses to COVID-19 mRNA vaccines in patients with solid tumors on active, immunosuppressive cancer therapy. *medRxiv — Preprint Server for Health Sciences* 2021.05.13.21257129.

Shulman, R. M., Weinberg, D. S., Ross, E. A., Ruth, K., Rall, G. F., Olszanski, A. J., et al. (2022). Adverse events reported by patients with cancer after administration of a 2-dose mRNA COVID-19 vaccine. *Journal of the National Comprehensive Cancer Network JNCCN, 20*(2), 160–166.

Singh, V., Dwivedi, S., Agrawal, R., Sadashiv, N., Fatima, G., & Abidi, A. (2024). The human monkeypox virus and host immunity: Emerging diagnostic and therapeutic challenges. *Infectious Disorders Drug Targets.*

Singhai, M., Das Gupta, G., Khurana, B., Arora, D., Ashique, S., & Mishra, N. (2024). Nanotechnology-based drug delivery systems for the treatment of cervical cancer: A comprehensive review. *Current Nanoscience, 20*(2), 224–247.

Suekane, S., Yutani, S., Yamada, A., Sasada, T., Matsueda, S., Takamori, S., et al. (2020). Identification of biomarkers for personalized peptide vaccination in 2,588 cancer patients. *International Journal of Oncology, 56*(6), 1479–1489.

Suschak, J. J., Williams, J. A., & Schmaljohn, C. S. (2017). Advancements in DNA vaccine vectors, non-mechanical delivery methods, and molecular adjuvants to increase immunogenicity. *Human Vaccines & Immunotherapeutics, 13*(12), 2837–2848.

Takada, N., Niwa, Y., Teshigawara, T., Isogai, K., Okura, H., & Matsuyama, A. (2020). The integrity of chemically treated plasmid DNA as a chemical-based choice for prion clearance. *Regenerative Therapy, 15*, 112–120.

Trimble, C. L., Morrow, M. P., Kraynyak, K. A., Shen, X., Dallas, M., Yan, J., et al. (2015). Safety, efficacy, and immunogenicity of VGX-3100, a therapeutic synthetic DNA vaccine targeting human papillomavirus 16 and 18 E6 and E7 proteins for cervical intraepithelial neoplasia 2/3: a randomised, double-blind, placebo-controlled phase 2b trial. *Lancet Lond Engl, 386*(10008), 2078–2088.

Van Lint, S., Wilgenhof, S., Heirman, C., Corthals, J., Breckpot, K., Bonehill, A., et al. (2014). Optimized dendritic cell-based immunotherapy for melanoma: The TriMix-formula. *Cancer Immunology, Immunotherapy CII, 63*(9), 959–967.

Ventola, C. L. (2017). Cancer immunotherapy, Part 3: Challenges and future trends. *Pharmacology & Therapeutics, 42*(8), 514–521.

Verbeke, R., Hogan, M. J., Loré, K., & Pardi, N. (2022). Innate immune mechanisms of mRNA vaccines. *Immunity, 55*(11), 1993–2005.

Vijayasingham, L., Bischof, E., & Wolfe, J. (2021). Gender and COVID-19 research agenda-setting initiative. Sex-disaggregated data in COVID-19 vaccine trials. *Lancet Lond Engl, 397*(10278), 966–967.

Villarreal, D. O., Talbott, K. T., Choo, D. K., Shedlock, D. J., & Weiner, D. B. (2013). Synthetic DNA vaccine strategies against persistent viral infections. *Expert Review of Vaccines, 12*(5), 537–554.

Vishweshwaraiah, Y. L., & Dokholyan, N. V. (2022). mRNA vaccines for cancer immunotherapy. *Frontiers in Immunology, 13*, 1029069.

Wang, B., Pei, J., Xu, S., Liu, J., & Yu, J. (2023b). Recent advances in mRNA cancer vaccines: meeting challenges and embracing opportunities. *Frontiers in Immunology, 14*, 1246682.

Wang, C., & Yuan, F. (2024). A comprehensive comparison of DNA and RNA vaccines. *Advanced Drug Delivery Reviews, 210*, 115340.

Wang, L. H., Wu, C. F., Rajasekaran, N., & Shin, Y. K. (2018). Loss of tumor suppressor gene function in human cancer: An overview. *Cellular Physiology & Biochemistry. International Journal of Experimental Cellular Physiology, Biochemistry and Pharmacology, 51*(6), 2647–2693.

Wang, Z., Jacobus, E. J., Stirling, D. C., Krumm, S., Flight, K. E., Cunliffe, R. F., et al. (2023a). Reducing cell intrinsic immunity to mRNA vaccine alters adaptive immune responses in mice. *Molecular Therapy Nucleic Acids, 34*, 102045.

Wilson, D. M., Duncton, M. A. J., Chang, C., Lee Luo, C., Georgiadis, T. M., Pellicena, P., et al. (2021). Early drug discovery and development of novel cancer therapeutics targeting DNA polymerase eta (POLH). *Frontiers in Oncology, 11*, 778925.

Witten, J., Hu, Y., Langer, R., & Anderson, D. G. (2024). Recent advances in nanoparticulate RNA delivery systems. *Proceedings of the National Academy of Sciences of the United States of America, 121*(11), e2307798120.

Wolff-Holz, E., & Weise, M. (2020). Biosimilars in the European Union: Current situation and challenges. *Bundesgesundheitsblatt, Gesundheitsforschung, Gesundheitsschutz, 63*(11), 1365–1372.

Wu, A., Zeng, Q., Kang, T. H., Peng, S., Roosinovich, E., Pai, S. I., et al. (2011). Innovative DNA vaccine for human papillomavirus (HPV)-associated head and neck cancer. *Gene Therapy, 18*(3), 304–312.

Xu, Q., Zhu, Y. F., Wang, H. C., Gong, Z. W., & Yu, Y. Z. (2016). Enhanced efficacy of DNA vaccination against botulinum neurotoxin serotype A by co-administration of plasmids encoding DC-stimulating Flt3L and MIP-3α cytokines. *Biologicals: Journal of the International Association of Biological Standardization, 44*(5), 441–447.

Xu, S., Yang, K., Li, R., & Zhang, L. (2020). mRNA vaccine era-mechanisms, drug platform and clinical prospection. *International Journal of Molecular Sciences, 21*(18), 6582.

Yao, R., Xie, C., & Xia, X. (2024). Recent progress in mRNA cancer vaccines. *Human Vaccines & Immunotherapeutics, 20*(1), 2307187.

Yousefi Adlsadabad, S., Hanrahan, J. W., & Kakkar, A. (2024). mRNA delivery: Challenges and advances through polymeric soft nanoparticles. *International Journal of Molecular Sciences, 25*(3), 1739.

Yuzhalin, A. E. (2024). Redefining cancer research for therapeutic breakthroughs. *British Journal of Cancer, 130*(7), 1078–1082.

Zhang, C., Maruggi, G., Shan, H., & Li, J. (2019). Advances in mRNA vaccines for infectious diseases. *Frontiers in Immunology, 10*, 594.

Zugazagoitia, J., Guedes, C., Ponce, S., Ferrer, I., Molina-Pinelo, S., & Paz-Ares, L. (2016). Current challenges in cancer treatment. *Clinical Therapeutics, 38*(7), 1551–1566.

CHAPTER TWO

Nucleic acid delivery as a therapeutic approach for cancer immunotherapy

Kashish Wilson[a], Garima[a], and Meenakshi Dhanawat[b],*

[a]M.M College of Pharmacy, Maharishi Markandeshwar (Deemed to be University), Mullana–Ambala, Haryana, India
[b]Amity Institute of Pharmacy, Amity University Haryana, Amity Education Valley, Panchgaon, Manesar, Gurugram, Haryana, India
*Corresponding author. e-mail address: meenakshi.itbhu@gmail.com; meenakshi.iitbhu@gmail.com

Contents

Abstract

The number of immuno-oncology medication approvals in current years has increased, indicating the immense potential of cancer immunotherapy. Nucleic acid therapy has advanced significantly in the interim. The diverse capabilities of nucleic acid therapies, gene-editing guide RNA (gRNA), immunomodulatory DNA/RNA, messenger RNA (mRNA), microRNA and siRNA, plasmids, and antisense oligonu-cleotides (ASO), for modification of immune responses and change the target endogenous or synthetic gene's expression, make them appealing. These skills can be extremely important in the creation of innovative immunotherapy approaches. To be effective, these treatments must, however, overcome a number of delivery challenges, such as quick in vivo disintegration, inadequate absorption inside target cells, necessary nuclear entrance, along with possible *in-vivo* toxic potential in tissues and cells that are healthy. Several of these obstacles have been addressed by the

ISSN 0065-2776, https://doi.org/10.1016/bs.ai.2024.10.009

development of nanoparticle delivery methods, which allow nucleic acid therapies to be safely and successfully delivered to immune cells. The nucleic acid applications for medicines employed for immunotherapy against cancer are covered in this chapter, along with the development of nanoparticle platforms that carry genome editing, mRNA, and DNA systems for improving the efficacy and safety profile in various therapies.

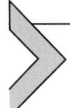

1. Introduction

1.1 Overview of cancer immunotherapy

To treat cancer patients, a new technique known as "cancer immunotherapy" utilizes immune system components. In this regard, certain therapeutic strategies involve the application of antibodies that attach to cancer cell-expressed proteins and inhibit them from completing their stated roles (Chen et al., 2020). Vaccinations, native T cell injections, as well as administration of immune cells that undergo genetic modification—like chimeric antigen receptor (CAR)-T cells or NK or CAR-T cells —are some instances of different tactics (Couzin-Frankel, 2013). Adoptive cell transfer of tumor-reactive T cells (ACT) regarded as highly effective therapy approach for hematological and solid tumors (Phan & Rosenberg, 2013). ACT enhances the potency of tumor cells, enabling them for to effective eradication of malignant cells in vivo. According to ACT recommendations, tumor-infiltrating lymphocytes (TILs) had been acquired, substantially established in vitro using cytokines to produce an appropriate frequency, and then implanted in the patient (Fan et al., 2018).

Currently, interest has grown for the application of chimeric antigen receptor (CAR)-based therapies, like CAR-NK cell and CAR-T cell, for specific targeting and elimination of tumor cells (Marofi et al., 2021b; Wang et al., 2017). The tumor microenvironment (TME) containing both natural killer (NK) cells and human T cells, which contributes considerably towards tumor immune monitoring. Prolonged, antigen-specific effector and memory immune responses are usually generated through T cells, while NK cells stimulate strong antitumor effects through the release of chemokines, cytokines associated with inflammation, and cytolytic complexes, which activate the immune systems, both innate and adaptive (Marofi et al., 2021a). Advances in cellular engineering technology have made it easier to genetically alter T and NK cells so they express CARs specific to tumor antigens (Altvater et al., 2009; Rosewell Shaw et al., 2017).

1.2 Role of nucleic acid in therapeutics

Immunotherapy and other nucleic acid treatments have emerged as potential options for cancer therapy (Opalinska & Gewirtz, 2002). An extensive variety of DNA or RNA known as nucleic acid treatments includes aptamers, gene-editing gRNA, mRNA, ASO, siRNA, miRNA, plasmids, and DNA and RNA immunomodulatory. The varying roles played by nucleic acid therapies include modulation (Pastor et al., 2018) of immune responses and gene expression regulation (up or down) Since 1995, there has been research on immunomodulatory nucleic acid (Sridharan & Gogtay, 2016), and an increasing number of prospective immunomodulatory nucleic acids are being found and investigated for application in immunotherapy (Fig. 1).

Nucleic acid therapies are regarded as affirmative possibilities for cancer immunotherapy because of their high specificity, adaptability, repeatable batch-to-batch manufacturing, and customizable immunogenicity. The five primary types of nucleic acid therapies regarding cancer immunotherapy will be covered in this article. Gene-regulating nucleic acid medications, like ASO as well as siRNA, may mute targeted genes and control post-transcriptional gene expression, therefore controlling the intracellular signaling cascade implicated for cancer formation (Dahlman et al., 2014). Immunostimulants including nucleic acids, like di-cyclic nucleotides which activate stimulator interferon genes (STING), can initiate or enhance anticancer immune stimulation, and poly I: C, 5′-triphosphate RNA, and unmethylated cytosine-guanosine deoxynucleotides (CpG) (Barber, 2015; Kyi et al., 2018; Vollmer & Krieg, 2009). It is possible to custom-design mRNA therapies and plasmid DNA (pDNA) for expressing specific peptides or proteins, like antigens or proteins utilized in

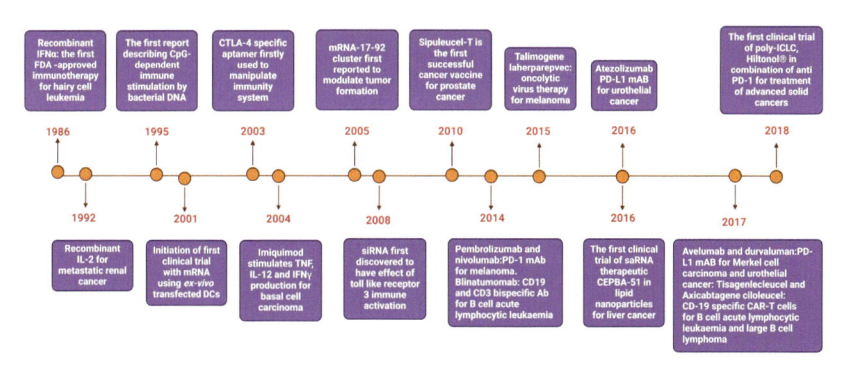

Fig. 1 Progress of immunomodulatory nucleic acids.

cancer immunotherapy (Hajj & Whitehead, 2017). Short single-stranded nucleic acids called aptamers undergo investigation as analogs of antibodies in nucleic acids in cancer immunotherapy (Gilboa et al., 2015). Lastly, nucleic acids related to genome editing, including gRNA, have recently been used to specifically modify targeted genes and subsequently modify Expression of genes promoting cancer immunotherapy (Yin et al., 2017). The successful and targeted transport of nucleic acid therapies into target areas within cells and tissues is essential leading to their widespread application (Fig. 2).

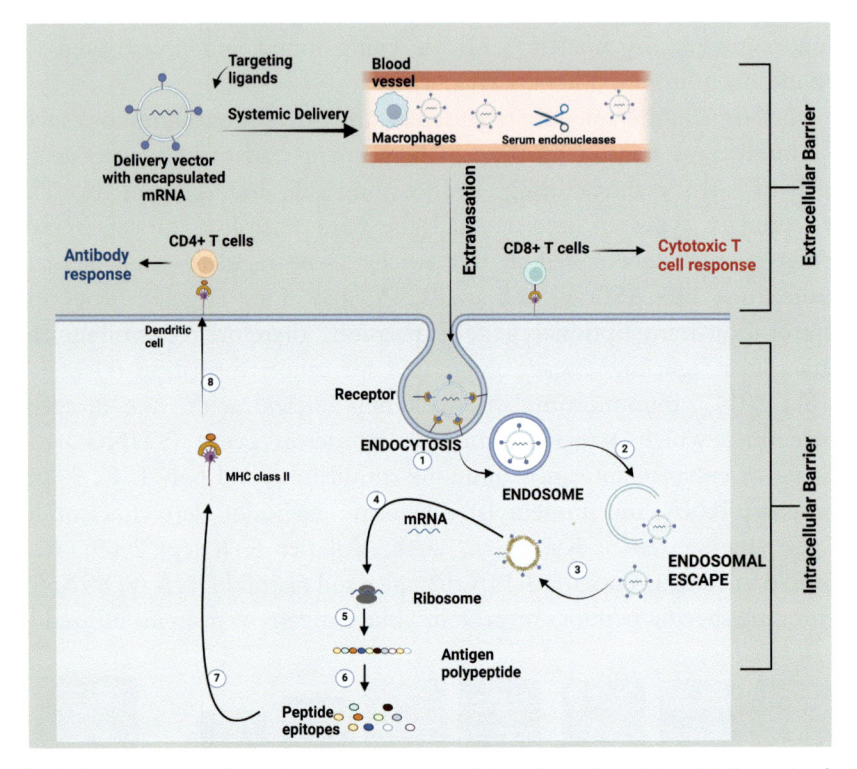

Fig. 2 Several major tissue-level targets in administration of nucleic acid therapies for cancer immunotherapy are the tumor microenvironment and lymphoid tissues. (A) Numerous cells, comprising tumor cells, antigen-presenting cells (DC, macrophage), lymphocytes (T cells, B cells, and NK cells), and fibroblasts, are found inside tumor microenvironment. These cells are essential for generation of tumor initiation, proliferation, and metastasis. (B) One of the intended locations for cancer therapies like vaccinations is the lymphatic system, which consists of the spleen and lymph nodes. Dendritic cells (DC), hepatocyte growth factor (HGF), myeloid-derived suppressor cells (MDSC), natural killer cells (NK cells), antigen-presenting cells (APCs), transforming growth factor-β (TGF-β), and matrix metalloproteinase (MMP).

Delivery of drug towards tumor cells is unmanageable due to complex tumor microenvironment (TME), that is additionally exacerbated through immunosuppression present inside TME. For example, TME provides high interstitial fluid pressure, acidosis, and tumor hypoxia. Additionally, stromal cells within TME, like cancer-associated fibroblasts (CAFs), which exaggerate HGF and TGF-β contribute for development of malignant tumors along with decrease in effectiveness of nucleic acid therapies when delivered in TME. Lymphoid tissues, which are home for various types of immune cells and are at areas of multitude of immune responses, are another significant category of tissue targets for immune treatment against cancer. For nucleic acid treatments, it is crucial to comprehend the delivery targets and develop delivery mechanisms appropriately. Nucleic acid treatments possess particular characteristics that may influence their distribution, unlike large biologics or standard small molecule medications. These characteristics include hydrophilic nature, negatively charged molecules, sensitivity to enzyme decomposition if left unmodified, and possibly undesired immunogenicity (Pack et al., 2005), plus the off-targeting impact (Verma & Somia, 1997). Numerous approaches have been developed throughout decades of research and development to solve these problems and further formation of various treatment for disease, like cancer immunotherapy (Pack et al., 2005). Nucleic acids can be chemically modified to increase their biostability by adding groups comparable to phosphorothioates to the backbone or 2′-F and 2′-O-methyl to the sugar (Brown & Suo, 2011; Egli & Manoharan, 2019). Furthermore, by creating steric hindrance that prevents nucleases from accessing nucleic acids, nanocarriers—which are frequently employed to transport therapeutic nucleic acids while safeguarding them from degradation by nuclease (Olton et al., 2007).

2. Delivery systems for nucleic acids

Gene therapy is a potentially effective treatment approach that involves delivering genes to treat various acute acquired and inherited disorders (Gillmore et al., 2021). Recently, a novel gene editing procedure called CRISPER has gained prominence through the use of Cas-encoding mRNA (Gillmore et al., 2021; Rosenblum et al., 2020). Due to the global coronavirus epidemic, mRNA has gained attention as a vaccine, and numerous businesses are developing more mRNA vaccines and therapies

(Jackson et al., 2020; Pardi et al., 2018). The initial vehicles for distributing protective genes, delivering therapeutic genes, and exploiting the viral life cycle were viruses (Ibraheem et al., 2014). Since viral vectors can effectively transfer genes and guarantee long-term expression, they are among the most commonly utilized gene therapy vectors (Nayerossadat et al., 2012).

Nucleic acids should be delivered to intracellular sites via convoluted routes for vaccinations and disease intervention to work. Nucleic acids encounter an array of challenging obstacles, such as the potential for negative immune responses (Shirley et al., 2020), the costly nature and challenges in their formation (Santos et al., 2020), and the little dimensions of genetic sequences which may be introduced inside human cells (Nagasaki & Shinkai, 2007). These obstacles eventually remain in the path of altering expression of protein by adding or substituting omitting or deficient genes, controlling gene expression using the level of RNA (e.g., silencing genes by RNA interference, alteration of RNA processing), regulating activity of microRNA, or by editing the genome and restructuring of cells. Therefore, therapy's clinical results have still not reached the expected levels of success, despite a wide spectrum of potential treatment techniques. The primary causes of systems for delivering genes failing in clinical trials are their absence of effectiveness along with problems relating to clinical security, particularly concerning viral vectors, that accounts for approximately 70% of gene therapy vectors (Fogel, 2018; Seyhan, 2019). As a result, non-viral strategies have emerged to address the shortcomings of viral systems. The safety benefits that non-viral systems provide above viral ones, the comparatively minimal reaction of the immune system, and the convenience of processing for permitting huge volumes at reduced revenue have drawn a lot of attention to this field of study (Gao et al., 2007).

Numerous non-viral vector systems enter the picture, including polymer supramolecular assemblies and liposomes, which have higher biological safety. However the main factor impeding their effectiveness is the therapeutic medicines' inadequate localization to the region of interest, both extracellularly and intracellularly (Blanco et al., 2015). Peptides provide excellent substitutes to get past these obstacles because of their exceptional potency, selectivity, and low toxicity (Muttenthaler et al., 2021). Furthermore, developments in nanosystems continue to pave the way for effective therapeutic delivery, making nanotechnology a preferred instrument in medicine (Blanco et al., 2015). Target cells internalize nanocarriers via a variety of mechanisms, including phagocytosis, micropinocytosis, cholesterol- or caveolae-mediated endocytosis, and clathrin-mediated endocytosis, depending on the surface's chemical science, size, charge, and shape (Kumari et al., 2010). Nanocarriers often stay sequestered in corresponding transport vesicles after entering cells through endocytosis; their fate is determined by both the endocytic pathway and the nanocarriers' physicochemical characteristics. Multiple membrane fusions are required for endosomal sequestration, whereby endocytic vesicles progressively fuse utilizing both delayed and initial endosomes before entering the lysosomal compartment. Throughout this pathway, a persistent drop in the intravesicular pH as well as rise in digestive enzyme composition having a significant effect on stability of payload and, consequently, efficacy (Parodi et al., 2015).

Due to these restrictions, methods for effectively shielding macromolecular medications from deterioration and precisely focusing on the main subcellular compartments are being sought after. Moreover, the necessity for carriers that can get past barriers in the site of delivery towards intracellular site of action is highlighted by an increase in discovery research aimed at improving our knowledge of intracellular trafficking routes (Petros & Desimone, 2010). The primary drawbacks of the most widely utilized non-viral methods of delivering nucleic acids, like polyplexes and lipoplexes, are their ineffective cytoplasmic delivery, nonspecific dispersion, as well as organelles focusing. Conversely, peptide-based nanocarriers, like peptide nanoparticles, are additionally referred to as peptiplexes, or peptidic multicompartment micelles, in addition to peptide-equipped nano-assemblies, have a lot of potential as delivery systems because they can be engineered to more easily penetrate cell membranes and localize to specific subcellular compartments. Peptides also have a desired bioactivity and are simple to synthesize. Because of their multivalent nature, the nanocarrier has a strong affinity towards the target (Ruoslahti, 2012). The potential to match peptides to target particular cells and tissues allows therapeutic nanocarriers to cross cell membrane and enter the desired target, resulting for improved intracellular dispersion and a prolonged therapeutic window (Jeong et al., 2018). Moreover, biocompatible nanocarriers and appropriate targeting moieties are just two of the promising solutions that smart delivery systems offer to address the uncontrolled release of payloads. These platforms also have stimulus-responsive components that enable triggered cargo release (Hossen et al., 2019). The idea that peptides can be used as targeting moieties for medical and analytical applications opened up innovative business opportunities in the pharma industry (Lee et al., 2019). Despite a modest pace of clinical advancement for peptides use, either by themselves or in conjunction using tiny components, significant funding, and extensive research endeavors attest to their auspicious potential as a therapeutic system delivery platform. This rare family of pharmaceutical compounds is in great demand due to increased interest in smart nanocarrier design, keeping an emphasis on cancer therapy among other things for precision medicine applications (Cooper et al., 2021; Mitchell et al., 2020; Sandra et al., 2019). Various delivery systems have been developed, each with its advantages and challenges shown in Table 1.

2.1 Delivery of nucleic acid therapeutics in cancer immunotherapy

Natural RNA can encode proteins, trigger innate immune responses, or modify the functionality of other proteins or RNAs, among other things (Pardi et al., 2018). mRNA transports genetic data transferred from DNA to the ribosome, which translates protein in the cytoplasm by using mRNA templates. mRNA treatments offer a great deal of potential for several applications, particularly cancer immunotherapy because mRNA can generate any proteins and peptides for a lengthy amount of time without demanding the localization of nuclear proteins for gene expression (Sahin et al., 2014). mRNA treatments avoid the possibility of permanent integration of genes within the genome, that leads to unfavorable side effects, as opposed to gene therapy which introduces genes to the human genome.

Nucleic acid chemistry has advanced to the point that it is now possible to create mRNA that is less immunogenic or resistant to enzyme breakdown. Multiple poly-A binding proteins (PABPs) can attach to the poly-A tail of endogenous mRNA in tandem enhancing the stability of mRNA and encouraging translation of mRNA (Wang et al., 1999). For mRNA vaccines, a poly-A tail of approximately 120 nucleotides continually improved the mRNA stability and translational effectiveness, offering a possible method for improving mRNA vaccines (Holtkamp et al., 2006). 5-methoxyuridine, N1-methylpseudouridine, and pseudouridine alterations in mRNA are additional chemical modification techniques that are successful in enhancing the stability of mRNA and enhancing protein expression (Li et al., 2016). A translation initiation nanoplex was created in the latest research by Li et al. It was composed of polyamine-loaded cationic carriers, eukaryotic initiation factor 4E (eIF4E) protein, and 7-methyguanosinecapped mRNA, which naturally recognize each other molecularly. The initial stage of protein synthesis can be imitated by these ribonucleoproteins (RNPs). They showed that the nanoplex improved

Table 1 Different delivery systems for nucleic acid therapies.

Delivery system	Characteristics	Advantages	Challenges
Polymer-Based Systems	Polymers that can form complexes with nucleic acids	DNA and RNA delivery, including gene editing	Variability in delivery efficiency, potential for toxicity
Viral Vectors	Engineered viruses that deliver nucleic acids into target cells	Gene therapy and CAR-T cell therapies	Risk of immune response and insertional mutagenesis
Exosomes	Naturally occurring vesicles that transport nucleic acids between cells	Delivery of therapeutic RNAs and proteins	Challenges in large-scale production and isolation
Lipid Nanoparticles (LNPs)	Nano-sized particles made of lipids that encapsulate nucleic acids	mRNA and siRNA delivery	Potential for toxicity and inflammation
Nanoparticles	Various materials (e.g., gold, silica)	Can be engineered for targeted delivery	Potential bioaccumulation, complex synthesis
Electroporation	Application of electrical pulses to introduce nucleic acids	Effective for local delivery, minimal invasiveness	Requires specialized equipment, potential tissue damage

mRNA stability, which improved mRNA transfection and increased cytotoxic CD8 T cell activation following stimulation of dendritic cells in mice (Li et al., 2017). Additionally, mRNA purification may decrease the innate immune system stimulation carried on via byproducts of mRNA treatments' synthesis (Karikó et al., 2011), which is how high-performance liquid chromatography (HPLC) is utilized for purifying mRNA in order to decrease the negative immunological response. Moreover, mRNA may currently be produced inexpensively and on a huge scale in vitro. Specifically, DNA templates, a phage RNA polymerase T7, T3, or Sp6 can be used to reliably synthesize mRNA using in vitro transcription (IVT). Using versatile techniques such as therapeutic adoptive cell engineering and ex vivo mRNA transfer and the direct use of cancer-specific mRNA vaccines that encode antigens specific to cancer, these technological breakthroughs have made mRNA treatments extremely promising for cancer immunotherapy (Sahin et al., 2014).

Undoubtedly, within the last ten years, the field of mRNA therapies has advanced remarkably. One such vaccination is RNActive®, which has been demonstrated to be absorbed through leukocytic cells and displayed by APCs for initiating adaptive immunity and immune cell activation (Sebastian et al., 2014). In the meantime, proinflammatory cytokine serum levels of immunized mice were not raised by these vaccines, indicating specificity for this mRNA vaccine, and only the injection and lymphoid sites exhibited stimulation of the immune system.

Double-stranded DNA (dsDNA) known as pDNA is made up of genes of interest and can be utilized in gene therapy to express target proteins or peptides or mRNA (Murakami & Sunada, 2011). The gene segment inside pDNA undergoes integration into the chromosomal genome to enable the persistent generation of protein or peptide products, and pDNA may replicate autonomously of chromosomal DNA. Research has already been conducted utilizing pDNA to generate RNA for muting target genes in cancer immunotherapy or to generate protein regulators (Liu et al., 2018; Luo et al., 2016; Song et al., 2018). Among the most widely used techniques for delivering pDNA is CaP NP because of its superior pH responsiveness, biocompatibility, and biodegradability (Qi et al., 2019). Olton et al. revealed that high transfection efficiencies were achieved by optimizing the Ca/P ratio and Ca2 + and PO43- solutions' technique for combining in CaP-pDNA nanoparticles (Olton et al., 2007). Targeting ligands were added to CaP lipid nanoparticles during further development to enable targeted distribution to cancer immunotherapy target cells (Luo & Liu, 2023; Qi et al., 2019).

To distribute pDNA encoding relaxin, Hu et al. created aminoethyl anisamide-modified lipid-CaP nanoparticles. This changed the stromal microenvironment and prevented colorectal, pancreatic, and breast cancer from metastasizing to the liver. Furthermore combined use of programmed death-ligand 1 (PD-L1) and relaxin-expression pDNA nanoparticles suppression enhanced the immunotherapeutic efficacy for this type of cancer model (Hu et al., 2019). For the transport of pDNA, polymer nanoparticles are also frequently employed. Liu et al. developed a copolymer known as LA-PegPI, which consists of PEI (molecular weight: ~800 Da), associated with Myo-inositol (INO), and coupled with a galactose-grafted PEG chain, to carry a pDNA that expresses interleukin-15 (IL-15) and tumor necrosis factor (TNF) by activating natural killer (NK) cells and CD8 + T lymphocytes. LAPegPI/pDNA therefore successfully stopped the growth of the tumor in the orthotopic hepatocellular cancer mouse model (Liu et al., 2018). However, because of their fragility and ineffective in vivo mRNA distribution, their usefulness has been restricted (Hajj & Whitehead, 2017). Effective in vivo delivery has many obstacles. mRNA vaccines need to elude renal clearance by glomerular filtration and prevent being broken down by the extracellular space and physiological fluids by endonucleases. To discharge mRNA to the cytosol, where translations occur, they must additionally permeate across the thick extracellular matrix before they reach the target cells (Zámečník et al., 2004), get picked up, and then escape the endosome.(Lorenz et al., 2011; Whitehead et al., 2009; Yin et al., 2014). These biological obstacles to in vivo mRNA administration have recently been addressed by delivery methods developed for this purpose (Fig. 3) (Oberli et al., 2017).

A new investigation created a lipid-based nanoparticle mRNA vaccination that targets dendritic cells exactly in vivo without requiring adhesion ligands or antibodies (Kranz et al., 2016). Several off-the-shelf lipids have been included in this platform, such as the zwitterionic lipid DOPE (1,2-dioleoyl-sn-glycero-3-phosphoethanolamine), the cationic lipids DOTMA (1,2-di-O-octa-decenyl-3-trimethylammonium-propane) and DOTAP (1,2-dioleoyl-3-trimethylammonium-propane) which create complexes with anionic mRNA (Ziller et al., 2018). It proved that changing the RNA–to-lipid ratio thus, in turn, the nanoparticle formulation surface charge enhanced intravenous mRNA that moves towards dendritic cell-comprising sections inside lymphoid organs and mouse spleen in addition to incorporating ligands or antibodies. It's important to note that in research utilizing nanoparticles with mRNA which produces a fluorescent protein, the whole biological distribution inside mice shows greater

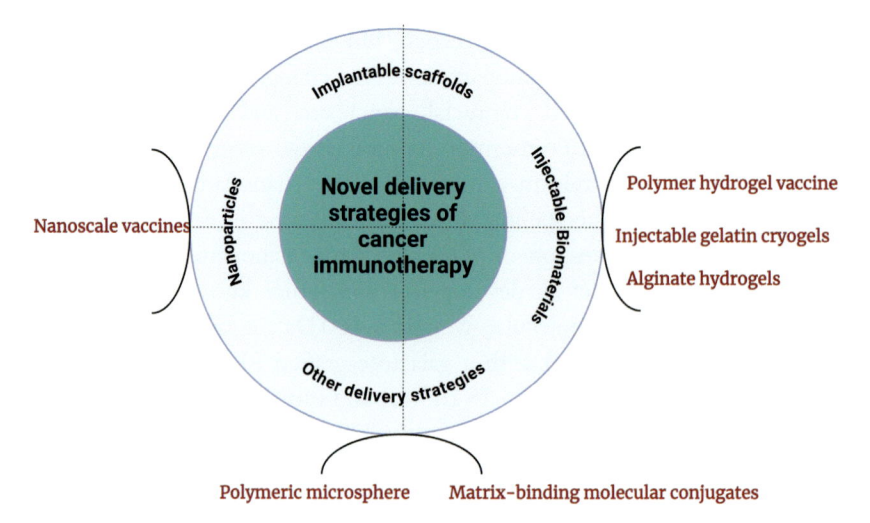

Fig. 3 Obstacles to dendritic cell delivery of the mRNA cancer vaccine. It can be done to develop an array of non-viral vectors that can transfer mRNA towards dendritic cells in vivo. These vectors must avoid themselves from being recognized by macrophages and prevent the mRNA from being taken down by serum endonucleases (this might be done by enclosing nucleic acids and altering their chemical makeup). Additionally, they have to prevent nonspecific interactions and renal clearance in the circulation (either by particle form or the use of polyethylene glycol, or PEG). Furthermore, in order to help dendritic cell entry and endosomal escape, these vectors should extravasate from the circulation and enter dendritic cells within target tissues. Following translation into the antigenic peptide in the cytosol, mRNA breaks down into small peptide epitopes that bind to either class I or class II molecules of the major histocompatibility complex (MHC). An antigen-specific antibody or cytotoxic T cell response occurs through MHCs' transmission of their antigenic epitopes to CD8 + (cytotoxic) or CD4 + (helper) T cells at the cell's surface. Sequential numbering shows the order in which the mRNA entrance and processing phases take place.

dependence on a charge of nanoparticle than the type of lipid quality employed. The potential lead nanoparticle allowed dendritic cells to read messenger RNA, produce tumor antigens, transport them to T cells, and drive robust tumor rejection in mouse models of lung, colorectal, and melanoma cancer (Kranz et al., 2016). Notably, this technology is undergoing clinical studies for the treatment of melanoma and has demonstrated encouraging patients' immunological responses.

2.2 Ionizable lipid nanoparticles for in vivo mRNA delivery

Cationic lipid-based methods are immunogenic and hazardous, despite their potentially effective results. Catalytic liposomes given intravenously possess a tendency to disrupt non-targeted cells' plasma membranes, damage the liver (Landesman-Milo & Peer, 2014), and lead to inflammation (Lv et al., 2006). Furthermore, anionic serum proteins can be adsorbed to liposomes to neutralize the lipids positive charge, which lowers the transport of nucleic acids inside cells (Ma et al., 2005). Ionizable lipid-like materials have been developed to circumvent difficulties associated with employing cationic lipids for mRNA-based immunotherapies. These materials lessen the harmful adverse reactions of cationic lipids while keeping their transfection qualities (Kauffman et al., 2015).

Ionizable lipids are less harmful than cationic lipids because, at physiological pH, they are neutral, but at low pH, they are positively charged, which renders them to bond with mRNA in nanoparticles inside acidic buffers (Kauffman et al., 2015). Lipids' positive charge amplifies cellular uptake by endocytosis, and when nanoparticles are deposited into endosomes, their pH drops (from around 6.8 to 4.5) as they change to become lysosomes (Scott et al., 2014). The theory suggests that ionizable lipids positive charge encourages electrostatic attraction as well as fusion of them with negatively charged endosomal membranes, resulting in bilayer destabilization and subsequently releasing of nucleic acids inside cytoplasm. Nevertheless, research is still being done to determine the exact mechanisms underlying endosomal release (Hafez et al., 2001; Walsh et al., 2013; Zelphati & Szoka, 1996).

A formulation of lipid nanoparticles consisting of cholesterol, phospholipid, ionizable lipid, and PEG–lipid conjugate was designed in a crucial study for delivering mRNA vaccines and triggering cytotoxic T-cell response. After being injected subcutaneously, the nanoparticles were able to infect several immune cells, like neutrophils, dendritic cells, and macrophages, they gathered in lymph nodes. In a melanoma mouse model, this technique was also assessed. Strong CD8 + T cell proliferation and functioning were elicited by a single immunization with nanoparticles, and animals given treatment with these nanoparticles lived longer in comparison to controls. Moreover, administering nanoparticles with mRNA expressing the tumor antigens gp100 (commonly known as PMEL) and TRP2 (commonly known as DCT) to mice in an invasive melanoma tumor model resulted in a wider reduction of the tumor as well as a rise in mortality. This study indicates ionizable lipid nanoparticles can boost mRNA vaccines dispersion as well as trigger significant immune system reactions (Hou et al., 2021).

Polymeric methods like dendrimers were additionally created for the administration of mRNA vaccines (Chahal et al., 2017). These methods are being utilized for delivering enormous medicinal payloads, like replicon mRNA, that can greatly boost the encoded protein synthesis. This was shown in several cases, such as vaccines against the Ebola virus, Toxoplasma gondii, and H1N1 influenza (Chahal et al., 2016). Thus, it is essential to evaluate these technologies' capability for delivering mRNA replicon for t continuous tumor antigens manufacturing.

3. Challenges in nucleic acid delivery

The capacity of nucleic acid medicines to operate efficiently and specifically distributed for targeting cells, tissues, and subcellular regions is essential for their widespread utilization. The complicated tumor micro-environment (TME), which gets worse by the immunosuppression asso-ciated with TME, makes drug delivery to tumor cells difficult. For example, TME possesses high interstitial fluid pressure, acidosis, and tumor hypoxia. Additionally, stromal cells within TME, like cancer-associated fibroblasts (CAFs), which exaggerate HGF and TGF-β, contributes for development of malignant tumors and decrease effectiveness of nucleic acid therapies when delivered inside TME (Li et al., 2007). Lymphoid tissues, which are home to various types of immune cells and are location of a multitude of immune responses, are another significant type of tissue target for immune therapy against cancer. For nucleic acid treatments, it is crucial to comprehend the delivery targets and develop delivery mechanisms appropriately. Nucleic acid therapeutics have particular characteristics that may influence their distribution, unlike big biologics or conventional small molecule medications. These characteristics include hydrophilic nature, negative charges, vulnerability to enzyme deterioration if left unaltered, potential undesirable immunogenicity (Pack et al., 2005), and off-targeting influence (Verma & Somia, 1997).

Due to their extreme instability, nucleic acids rapidly break down nucleases occurrence besides entering targeted tissues (Kauffman et al., 2016). Furthermore, nucleic acids cannot pass cells on their own; instead, physical methods (such as electroporation) or transfection chemicals are needed, both of which are impractical for use in vivo and extremely harmful to cells when used in ex vivo (Moffett et al., 2017; Stewart et al., 2016). Another delivery challenge for many nucleic acid therapies, including DNA and gene editing components, is getting past the nuclear membrane so they can be reproduced inside nucleus (McNamara et al., 2015). Therefore, to entirely understand the substantial therapeutic efficacy of the molecules, there is a significant deal of interest in creating innovative delivery options that can both enclose and preserve nucleic acids and facilitate their distribution within the targeted cells and tissues.

Numerous approaches have been developed throughout decades of research and development to solve these problems and further the formation of nucleic acid therapies in the therapy of disease, including cancer immunotherapy (Hajj & Whitehead, 2017; Pack et al., 2005). Chemical modification of nucleic acids, such as adding 2′-Oand 2′-F-methyl to the backbone of the sugar or phosphorothioate, is a frequently employed tactic to increase the biostability of nucleic acids (Brown & Suo, 2011; Egli & Manoharan, 2019). Furthermore, by creating steric hindrance that prevents nucleases from accessing nucleic acids, nanocarriers— which are commonly used for transporting therapeutic nucleic acids—can protect nucleic acids from breakdown by nuclease (Olton et al., 2007).

4. Recent advances in delivery technologies

Utilizing T-cells to administer treatments and other cutting-edge biomaterials and drug delivery techniques like nanoparticles could efficiently harness immunotherapies, increase their efficacy, and lessen their harmful side effects. Vaccine delivery can be mediated by nanoparticles (Fig. 4).

Antigen (such as peptides and proteins)-TLR agonist fusion vaccines were the most studied type of nanoscale vaccinations (Ignacio et al., 2018; Xu & Moyle, 2018). The adjuvant and antigen can be codelivered to the same immune cell when TLR agonists and antigen are combined. TLR7/8 agonists were linked with polymer scaffolds in a representative work, which also showed that polymer-TLR7/8 agonists may assemble themselves to particles having a diameter of 10–20 nm when the agonist density is low. In comparison with unformulated TLR7/8 agonists, the lymph nodes released more cytokines (Lynn et al., 2015). Additionally, amphiphilic vaccinations at the nanoscale made of adjuvant or antigen payload connected to the lipophilic albumin's tail have been developed (Liu et al., 2014).

When administered in vivo, these nano-vaccines have the potential to greatly concentrate in lymph nodes and decrease systemic dispersion. The outcomes demonstrated a thirty-fold increase in T cell activation, a

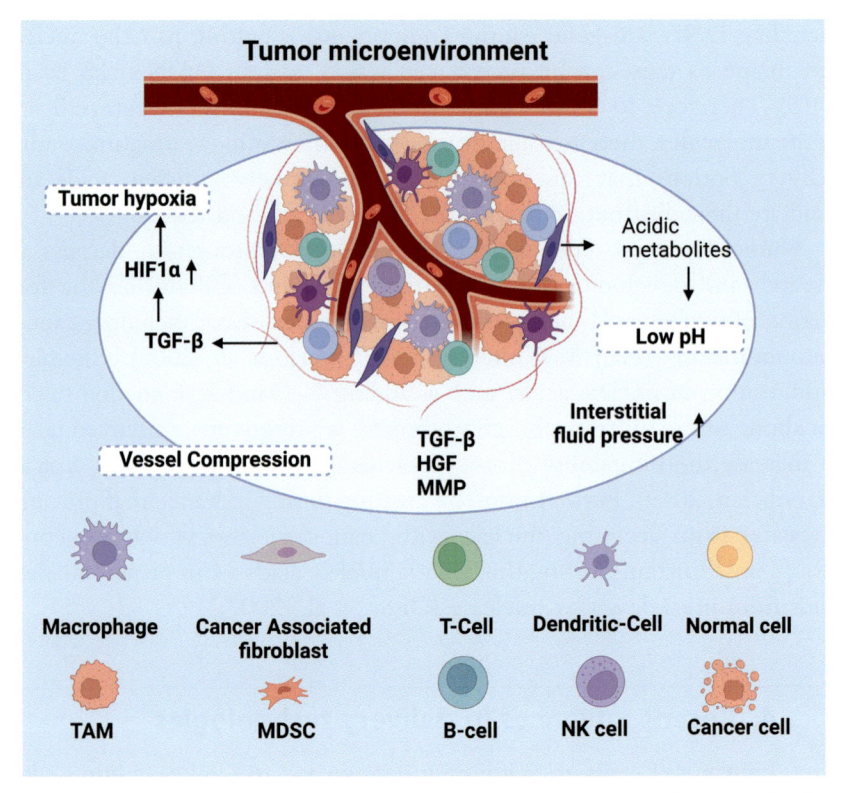

Fig. 4 Novel delivery strategies of immunotherapy with improved efficacy and safety.

substantial enhancement of immune response against tumors, and a significant reduction in systemic toxicity. This easy-to-implement delivery method boosts the vaccine's safety and effectiveness simultaneously. Furthermore, neoantigen peptide and adjuvant-conjugated high-density lipoprotein mimic nanodiscs were created (Kuai et al., 2016). Vaccines based on nanodiscs can significantly improve the effectiveness of adjuvant and antigen co-delivery to lymphoid tissues, maintaining antigen presentation to DCs. Nanodiscs often elicit neoantigen-specific immune responses at a frequency as high as 40 times higher than soluble vaccines. When anti-PD-1 as well as anti-CTLA-4 medication undergoes pairing among nanodiscs, tumors in animal models were eradicated (Hafez et al., 2001). As a result, the vaccination based on nanodiscs holds promise for tailored cancer immunotherapy. A range of current and emerging technologies are utilized to ensure the efficacious as well as target delivery of these therapeutics to cancer cells shown in Table 2.

Table 2 Current and emerging technologies for nucleic acid delivery.

Technology	Description	Advantages	Challenges
CRISPR/Cas9	Gene-editing technology that can modify DNA sequences	High precision, potential for permanent effects	Ethical concerns, off-target effects
Adeno-Associated Virus (AAV) Vectors	Vectors obtained through AAV that deliver genetic material to target cells	Low immunogenicity, long-term expression	Limited capacity for large genes, high production costs
Nanoplexes	Nanoscale complexes formed by nucleic acids and targeting ligands	High versatility, can be tailored for specific targets	Potential toxicity, complex formulation processes

4.1 Implantable scaffolds for immunotherapy

Implantable scaffolds are regarded as biomaterials which could be reloaded from an array of chemical reagents, biological agents, or cells. Usually, a brief surgical procedure is used to implant the scaffolds into the resected or subcutaneous areas. The implants' dimensions are in line with those of a little tablet or pill. The released bioactive substances within the implanted scaffold can be regulated, and immune cells are usually attracted to scaffolds to access them for additional bio-programming (Koshy & Mooney, 2016; Leifer, 2017). Poly (lactide-co-glycolide) (PLG) polymer scaffolds have been enriched from tumor cell lysates and GM-CSF, CpG oligonucleotides, as recruitment factors, hazard signals, and antigen reports, in that sequence. Populations of dendritic cells may be chosen and educated in specific ways (Ali et al., 2009). The implanted scaffold might remain inside human body for a period greater than a week for effective stimulation of immune system and stop the tumor from developing. It has been shown in brain tumor models that the anti-tumor effect of the implant is immensely associated with its capacity to enter tumor tissue site and form gradient of GM-CSF (Ali et al., 2011).

PLG scaffolds are mainly designed for their utilization in innovative ways for delivering a range of agonists. Additionally, ICIs and scaffolds together may increase CTL activity. At present, a phase I clinical investigation is evaluating the WDVAX vaccine (ClinicalTrials.gov identifier: NCT01753089) inside individuals diagnosed from melanoma stage IV

(Xie et al., 2023). Immense anticipation describes that targeted antigens or artificial neoantigens might create create customized vaccinations (Kim et al., 2014).

4.2 Injectable biomaterials for immunotherapy

Biomaterials that can be administered include hydrogels and cryogels (Hixon et al., 2017). These materials have the advantage of not requiring surgical implantation; they can be positioned wherever the needle may go. This is low-risk, minimally intrusive method that doesn't require a lot of technical know-how and can prevent needless tissue damage as well as a number of issues linked to an inflammatory wound response (Koshy et al., 2014). To enhance DC penetration and immunological reprogramming, injectable polymer hydrogel vaccines were developed as immune initiation centers. Additionally, hydrogels were packed with chemoattractants and immunomodulators. Injectable treatment doubled the survival rate of models for B cell lymphoma (Singh et al., 2011). Later, a combination of hydrogel along with microsphere with two layers was created to transport exogenous immune cells. A hydrogel that could carry exogenous DCs was created in situ using an injectable alginate-based method (Hori et al., 2008). It also investigated whether immunostimulatory chemicals could be delivered via encapsulation in bulk using a self-gelling apparatus. Cryogels of injectable gelatin derived from natural collagen have been shown in recent years to regulate the release of GM-CSF and promote immune cell infiltration and growth. Furthermore, the alginate hydrogel system was applied to generate pores which were larger compared to those of the traditional nanoporous alginate systems (Verbeke & Mooney, 2015). When injected with GM-CSF, the macroporous alginate hydrogels significantly enhanced cell penetration and attracted millions of immature DCs to the region. Further research has demonstrated that physically conjugated peptide antigens could be carried through identical pore-forming alginate hydrogels loaded with GM-CSF, forming the acquisition as well as activation of antigen-specific T lymphocytes (Verbeke et al., 2017).

4.3 Other delivery strategies: matrix-binding molecular conjugates, mineral oils, and polymeric microspheres

To decrease systemic medication exposure and side effects, tumors may build up within and around matrix-binding molecular conjugates. For example, checkpoint inhibitors utilize a water-soluble amine-sulfhydryl crosslinker to attach to the peptide of placental growth factor 2 (PLGF2), having enhanced affinity for an array of matrix proteins. In respect to mice models of breast cancer as well as melanoma, many conjugates became extensively localized inside cells matrix surrounding the tumor tissue after peritumoral injection than those of the unaltered antagonists., which caused the development of the tumor to get delayed and lifespan to rise (Ishihara et al., 2017). These conjugates also reduced side effects associated with systemic ICI therapy and increased systemic anti-tumor immunity. Furthermore, because of the scalable nature of the matrix-binding molecular conjugate, ICIs can be locally delivered to various body tumor sites that are challenging to reach through systemic administration.

5. Conclusion

Nucleic acid therapy's potential for treating a wide range of ailments has never been seen before. There is a lot of interest in using nucleic acid treatments for cancer immunotherapy because of recent developments in immuno-oncology and nucleic acid therapeutics. Therapeutics involving nucleic acids offer an enormous span of applications. Nucleic acid treatments, including immunomodulatory nucleic acids, pDNA and mRNA therapeutics, and gene-regulating nucleic acid medications (gRNA, siRNA, ASO, etc.) utilize the ability for gene expression manipulation and subsequently regulate protein activities to modify immune responses. Because of their inherent negative charges, enzymatic degradation vulnerability, and quick bodily clearance, natural nucleic acids may not be as effective as they could be in clinical settings. Furthermore, numerous physiological barriers provide significant obstacles to the effective distribution of drugs containing nucleic acids to the intended tissues, cells, and subcellular locations. To effectively be absorbed by tumor-associated cells, systemically delivered tumor-targeted nucleic acid medications, for example, might be able to pass through blood vessel endothelium barriers before entering the tumor's milieu. Regarding nucleic acid medications that boost immune responses, it is intended for these medications to build up in immune cells as well as lymphoid tissues to increase the lymphocyte's capacity to infiltrate tumors. Finally, about nucleic acid treatments that function inside cytoplasm or even inside nuclei, enhancing endosome release throughout endocytosis-mediated absorption of cells is crucial. For example, cytosolic delivery of mRNA therapeutics is required for translating peptides or proteins, adjuvants which leads to stimulation of immune system according to cytosolic nucleic acid detection, like STING agonists, additionally anticipated; and nuclei are the usual intracellular locations of pDNA and nucleic acids that alter the genome. Several chemical alterations in nucleic acids and drug delivery methods have been created, which are effective in addressing these issues by enhancing the drugs' tissue and cell delivery, pharmacokinetics, and biostability. Utilizing nucleic acid chemistry, numerous chemical changes have been developed for the nucleosides, sugar, and support for empowering the treatment effectiveness as well as biostability, reducing negative adverse impact, and off-targeting. Furthermore, a range of drug delivery methods have been documented via the administration of treatments using nucleic acids for tissues and cells. Nanoparticles of lipids, polymers, viruses, and bioconjugates are examples of representative delivery mechanisms for nucleic acid treatments; however, these were outside the purview of this article's discussion. Nucleic acid treatments offer potential, as evidenced by the approval of several siRNA by the US FDA recently for liver ailments therapies employing Lipid nanoparticles or bioconjugates of GalNAc. It is intended that future research focus on creating therapies with nucleic acids— encompassing methods of delivery— for tissues and organs outside the liver in order to cure diseases like cancer through immunotherapy. Furthermore, it is anticipated that developments in ASO and siRNA therapeutics may spur the creation of further oligonucleotide therapies, including gRNA and microRNA. Finally, the creation of more therapies using nucleic acids, particularly frequently big mRNA, should benefit from the expertise gained within the pDNA therapies domain. In order to deal with issues with current immunotherapy approaches, including an inability to overcome blocking immune checkpoints and a typically inadequate response rate, it is anticipated that the creation of new nucleic acid treatments and their delivery systems will prove crucial for enhancing results during the immune therapy of cancer. This is a result of a growing reservoir of information concerning immuno-oncology pathways.

References

Ali, O. A., Doherty, E., Mooney, D. J., & Emerich, D. (2011). Relationship of vaccine efficacy to the kinetics of DC and T-cell responses induced by PLG-based cancer vaccines. *Biomatter, 1*, 66–75.

Ali, O. A., Emerich, D., Dranoff, G., & Mooney, D. J. (2009). In situ regulation of DC subsets and T cells mediates tumor regression in mice. *Science Translational Medicine, 1*, 8ra19.

Altvater, B., Landmeier, S., Pscherer, S., Temme, J., Schweer, K., Kailayangiri, S., ... Rossig, C. (2009). 2B4 (CD244) signaling by recombinant antigen-specific chimeric receptors costimulates natural killer cell activation to leukemia and neuroblastoma cells. *Clinical Cancer Research: An Official Journal of the American Association for Cancer Research, 15*, 4857–4866.

Barber, G. N. (2015). STING: Infection, inflammation and cancer. *Nature Reviews. Immunology, 1512*(15), 760–770 2015.

Blanco, E., Shen, H., & Ferrari, M. (2015). Principles of nanoparticle design for overcoming biological barriers to drug delivery. *Nature Biotechnology, 339*(33), 941–951 2015.

Brown, J. A., & Suo, Z. (2011). Unlocking the sugar "steric gate" of DNA polymerases. *Biochemistry, 50*, 1135–1142.

Chahal, J. S., Fang, T., Woodham, A. W., Khan, O. F., Ling, J., Anderson, D. G., & Ploegh, H. L. (2017). An RNA nanoparticle vaccine against Zika virus elicits antibody and CD8+ T cell responses in a mouse model. *Scientific Reports, 7*, 1–9 2017 71.

Chahal, J. S., Khan, O. F., Cooper, C. L., McPartlan, J. S., Tsosie, J. K., Tilley, L. D., ... Anderson, D. G. (2016). Dendrimer-RNA nanoparticles generate protective immunity against lethal Ebola, H1N1 influenza, and Toxoplasma gondii challenges with a single dose. *Proceedings of the National Academy of Sciences of the United States of America, 113*, E4133–E4142.

Chen, W., Yuan, Y., & Jiang, X. (2020). Antibody and antibody fragments for cancer immunotherapy. *Journal of Controlled Release: Official Journal of the Controlled Release Society, 328*, 395–406.

Cooper, B. M., Iegre, J., O'Donovan, D. H., Ölwegård Halvarsson, M., & Spring, D. R. (2021). Peptides as a platform for targeted therapeutics for cancer: Peptide–drug conjugates (PDCs). *Chemical Society Reviews, 50*, 1480–1494.

Couzin-Frankel, J. (2013). Breakthrough of the year 2013. Cancer immunotherapy. *Science (New York, N. Y.), 342*, 1432–1433.

Dahlman, J. E., Barnes, C., Khan, O. F., Thiriot, A., Jhunjunwala, S., Shaw, T. E., ... Anderson, D. G. (2014). In vivo endothelial siRNA delivery using polymeric nanoparticles with low molecular weight. *Nature Nanotechnology, 98*(9), 648–655 2014.

Egli, M., & Manoharan, M. (2019). Re-engineering RNA molecules into therapeutic agents. *Accounts of Chemical Research, 52*, 1036–1047.

Fan, J., Shang, D., Han, B., Song, J., Chen, H., & Yang, J. M. (2018). Adoptive cell transfer: Is it a promising immunotherapy for colorectal cancer? *Theranostics, 8*, 5784.

Fogel, D. B. (2018). Factors associated with clinical trials that fail and opportunities for improving the likelihood of success: A review. *Contemporary Clinical Trials Communications, 11*, 156.

Gao, X., Kim, K. S., & Liu, D. (2007). Nonviral gene delivery: What we know and what is next. *The AAPS Journal, 9*.

Gilboa, E., Berezhnoy, A., & Schrand, B. (2015). Reducing toxicity of immune therapy using aptamer-targeted drug delivery. *Cancer Immunology Research, 3*, 1195–1200.

Gillmore, J. D., Gane, E., Taubel, J., Kao, J., Fontana, M., Maitland, M. L., ... Lebwohl, D. (2021). CRISPR-Cas9 in vivo gene editing for transthyretin amyloidosis. *The New England Journal of Medicine, 385*, 493–502.

Hafez, I. M., Maurer, N., & Cullis, P. R. (2001). On the mechanism whereby cationic lipids promote intracellular delivery of polynucleic acids. *Gene Therapy, 815*(8), 1188–1196 2001.

Hajj, K. A., & Whitehead, K. A. (2017). Tools for translation: Non-viral materials for therapeutic mRNA delivery. *Nature Reviews Materials, 210*(2), 1–17 2017.

Hixon, K. R., Lu, T., & Sell, S. A. (2017). A comprehensive review of cryogels and their roles in tissue engineering applications. *Acta Biomaterialia, 62*, 29–41.

Holtkamp, S., Kreiter, S., Selmi, A., Simon, P., Koslowski, M., Huber, C., ... Sahin, U. (2006). Modification of antigen-encoding RNA increases stability, translational efficacy, and T-cell stimulatory capacity of dendritic cells. *Blood, 108,* 4009–4017.

Hori, Y., Winans, A. M., Huang, C. C., Horrigan, E. M., & Irvine, D. J. (2008). Injectable dendritic cell-carrying alginate gels for immunization and immunotherapy. *Biomaterials, 29,* 3671–3682.

Hossen, S., Hossain, M. K., Basher, M. K., Mia, M. N. H., Rahman, M. T., & Uddin, M. J. (2019). Smart nanocarrier-based drug delivery systems for cancer therapy and toxicity studies: A review. *Journal of Advanced Research, 15,* 1–18.

Hou, X., Zaks, T., Langer, R., & Dong, Y. (2021). Lipid nanoparticles for mRNA delivery. *Nature Reviews Materials, 612*(6), 1078–1094 2021.

Hu, M., Wang, Y., Xu, L., An, S., Tang, Y., Zhou, X., ... Huang, L. (2019). Relaxin gene delivery mitigates liver metastasis and synergizes with check point therapy. *Nature Communications, 101*(10), 1–13 2019.

Ibraheem, D., Elaissari, A., & Fessi, H. (2014). Gene therapy and DNA delivery systems. *International Journal of Pharmaceutics, 459,* 70–83.

Ignacio, B. J., Albin, T. J., Esser-Kahn, A. P., & Verdoes, M. (2018). Toll-like receptor agonist conjugation: A chemical perspective. *Bioconjugate Chemistry, 29,* 587–603.

Ishihara, J., Fukunaga, K., Ishihara, A., Larsson, H. M., Potin, L., Hosseinchi, P., ... Hubbell, J. A. (2017). Matrix-binding checkpoint immunotherapies enhance antitumor efficacy and reduce adverse events. *Science Translational Medicine, 9.*

Jackson, L. A., Anderson, E. J., Rouphael, N. G., Roberts, P. C., Makhene, M., Coler, R. N., ... Beigel, J. H. (2020). An mRNA vaccine against SARS-CoV-2—Preliminary report. *The New England Journal of Medicine, 383,* 1920–1931.

Jeong, W. J., Bu, J., Kubiatowicz, L. J., Chen, S. S., Kim, Y. S., & Hong, S. (2018). Peptide–nanoparticle conjugates: A next generation of diagnostic and therapeutic platforms? *Nano Convergence, 51*(5), 1–18 2018.

Karikó, K., Muramatsu, H., Ludwig, J., & Weissman, D. (2011). Generating the optimal mRNA for therapy: HPLC purification eliminates immune activation and improves translation of nucleoside-modified, protein-encoding mRNA. *Nucleic Acids Research, 39.*

Kauffman, K. J., Dorkin, J. R., Yang, J. H., Heartlein, M. W., Derosa, F., Mir, F. F., ... Anderson, D. G. (2015). Optimization of lipid nanoparticle formulations for mRNA delivery in vivo with fractional factorial and definitive screening designs. *Nano Letters, 15,* 7300–7306.

Kauffman, K. J., Webber, M. J., & Anderson, D. G. (2016). Materials for non-viral intracellular delivery of messenger RNA therapeutics. *Journal of Controlled Release: Official Journal of the Controlled Release Society, 240,* 227–234.

Kim, J., Li, W. A., Choi, Y., Lewin, S. A., Verbeke, C. S., Dranoff, G., & Mooney, D. J. (2014). Injectable, spontaneously assembling, inorganic scaffolds modulate immune cells in vivo and increase vaccine efficacy. *Nature Biotechnology, 331*(33), 64–72 2014.

Koshy, S. T., Ferrante, T. C., Lewin, S. A., & Mooney, D. J. (2014). Injectable, porous, and cell-responsive gelatin cryogels. *Biomaterials, 35,* 2477–2487.

Koshy, S. T., & Mooney, D. J. (2016). Biomaterials for enhancing anti-cancer immunity. *Current Opinion in Biotechnology, 40,* 1.

Kranz, L. M., Diken, M., Haas, H., Kreiter, S., Loquai, C., Reuter, K. C., ... Sahin, U. (2016). Systemic RNA delivery to dendritic cells exploits antiviral defence for cancer immunotherapy. *Nature, 5347607*(534), 396–401 2016.

Kuai, R., Ochyl, L. J., Bahjat, K. S., Schwendeman, A., & Moon, J. J. (2016). Designer vaccine nanodiscs for personalized cancer immunotherapy. *Nature Materials, 164*(16), 489–496 2017.

Kumari, S., Mg, S., & Mayor, S. (2010). Endocytosis unplugged: Multiple ways to enter the cell. *Cell Research, 203*(20), 256–275 2010.

Kyi, C., Roudko, V., Sabado, R., Saenger, Y., Loging, W., Mandeli, J., ... Bhardwaj, N. (2018). Therapeutic immune modulation against solid cancers with intratumoral poly-ICLC: A pilot trial. *Clinical Cancer Research: An Official Journal of the American Association for Cancer Research, 24*, 4937–4948.

Landesman-Milo, D., & Peer, D. (2014). Toxicity profiling of several common RNAi-based nanomedicines: A comparative study. *Drug Delivery and Translational Research, 4*, 96–103.

Lee, A. C. L., Harris, J. L., Khanna, K. K., & Hong, J. H. (2019). A comprehensive review on current advances in peptide drug development and design. *International Journal of Molecular Sciences, 20*.

Leifer, C. A. (2017). Dendritic cells in host response to biologic scaffolds. *Seminars in Immunology, 29*, 41–48.

Li, B., Luo, X., & Dong, Y. (2016). Effects of chemically modified messenger RNA on protein expression. *Bioconjugate Chemistry, 27*, 849–853.

Li, H., Fan, X., & Houghton, J. M. (2007). Tumor microenvironment: The role of the tumor stroma in cancer. *Journal of Cellular Biochemistry, 101*, 805–815.

Li, J., Wang, W., He, Y., Li, Y., Yan, E. Z., Zhang, K., ... Hammond, P. T. (2017). Structurally programmed assembly of translation initiation nanoplex for superior mRNA delivery. *ACS Nano, 11*, 2531–2544.

Liu, H., Moynihan, K. D., Zheng, Y., Szeto, G. L., Li, A. V., Huang, B., ... Irvine, D. J. (2014). Structure-based programming of lymph-node targeting in molecular vaccines. *Nature, 5077493*(507), 519–522 2014.

Liu, L., Zong, Z. M., Liu, Q., Jiang, S. S., Zhang, Q., Cen, L. Q., ... Yao, H. (2018). A novel galactose-PEG-conjugated biodegradable copolymer is an efficient gene delivery vector for immunotherapy of hepatocellular carcinoma. *Biomaterials, 184*, 20–30.

Liu, Q., Zhu, H., Tiruthani, K., Shen, L., Chen, F., Gao, K., ... Huang, L. (2018). Nanoparticle-mediated trapping of Wnt family member 5A in tumor microenvironments enhances immunotherapy for B-Raf proto-oncogene mutant melanoma. *ACS Nano, 12*, 1250–1261.

Lorenz, C., Fotin-Mleczek, M., Roth, G., Becker, C., Dam, T. C., Verdurmen, W. P. R., ... Schlake, T. (2011). Protein expression from exogenous mRNA: Uptake by receptor-mediated endocytosis and trafficking via the lysosomal pathway. *RNA Biology, 8*.

Luo, C., Miao, L., Zhao, Y., Musetti, S., Wang, Y., Shi, K., & Huang, L. (2016). A novel cationic lipid with intrinsic antitumor activity to facilitate gene therapy of TRAIL DNA. *Biomaterials, 102*, 239–248.

Luo, Z., & Liu, X. (2023). Nanomaterials for cancer immunotherapy, what is the next? *Next Nanotechnology, 1*, 100006.

Lv, H., Zhang, S., Wang, B., Cui, S., & Yan, J. (2006). Toxicity of cationic lipids and cationic polymers in gene delivery. *Journal of Controlled Release: Official Journal of the Controlled Release Society, 114*, 100–109.

Lynn, G. M., Laga, R., Darrah, P. A., Ishizuka, A. S., Balaci, A. J., Dulcey, A. E., ... Seder, R. A. (2015). In vivo characterization of the physicochemical properties of polymer-linked TLR agonists that enhance vaccine immunogenicity. *Nature Biotechnology, 3311*(33), 1201–1210 2015.

Ma, Z., Li, J., He, F., Wilson, A., Pitt, B., & Li, S. (2005). Cationic lipids enhance siRNA-mediated interferon response in mice. *Biochemical and Biophysical Research Communications, 330*, 755–759.

Marofi, F., Abdul-Rasheed, O. F., Rahman, H. S., Budi, H. S., Jalil, A. T., Yumashev, A. V., ... Jarahian, M. (2021a). CAR-NK cell in cancer immunotherapy; A promising frontier. *Cancer Science, 112*, 3427.

Marofi, F., Motavalli, R., Safonov, V. A., Thangavelu, L., Yumashev, A. V., Alexander, M., ... Khiavi, F. M. (2021b). CAR T cells in solid tumors: Challenges and opportunities. *Stem Cell Research & Therapy, 121*(12), 1–16 2021.

McNamara, M. A., Nair, S. K., & Holl, E. K. (2015). RNA-based vaccines in cancer immunotherapy. *Journal of Immunology Research, 2015*.

Mitchell, M. J., Billingsley, M. M., Haley, R. M., Wechsler, M. E., Peppas, N. A., & Langer, R. (2020). Engineering precision nanoparticles for drug delivery. *Nature Reviews. Drug Discovery, 202*(20), 101–124 2020.

Moffett, H. F., Coon, M. E., Radtke, S., Stephan, S. B., McKnight, L., Lambert, A., ... Stephan, M. T. (2017). Hit-and-run programming of therapeutic cytoreagents using mRNA nanocarriers. *Nature Communications, 8*.

Murakami, T., & Sunada, Y. (2011). Plasmid DNA gene therapy by electroporation: Principles and recent advances. *Current Gene Therapy, 11*, 447–456.

Muttenthaler, M., King, G. F., Adams, D. J., & Alewood, P. F. (2021). Trends in peptide drug discovery. *Nature Reviews. Drug Discovery, 204*(20), 309–325 2021.

Nagasaki, T., & Shinkai, S. (2007). The concept of molecular machinery is useful for design of stimuli-responsive gene delivery systems in the mammalian cell. *Journal of Inclusion Phenomena and Macrocyclic Chemistry, 583*(58), 205–219 2007.

Nayerossadat, N., Maedeh, T., & Ali, P. A. (2012). Viral and nonviral delivery systems for gene delivery. *Advanced Biomedical Research, 1*, 27.

Oberli, M. A., Reichmuth, A. M., Dorkin, J. R., Mitchell, M. J., Fenton, O. S., Jaklenec, A., ... Blankschtein, D. (2017). Lipid nanoparticle assisted mRNA delivery for potent cancer immunotherapy. *Nano Letters, 17*, 1326–1335.

Olton, D., Li, J., Wilson, M. E., Rogers, T., Close, J., Huang, L., ... Sfeir, C. (2007). Nanostructured calcium phosphates (NanoCaPs) for non-viral gene delivery: Influence of the synthesis parameters on transfection efficiency. *Biomaterials, 28*, 1267–1279.

Opalinska, J. B., & Gewirtz, A. M. (2002). Nucleic-acid therapeutics: Basic principles and recent applications. *Nature Reviews. Drug Discovery, 17*(1), 503–514.

Pack, D. W., Hoffman, A. S., Pun, S., & Stayton, P. S. (2005). Design and development of polymers for gene delivery. *Nature Reviews. Drug Discovery, 47*(4), 581–593.

Pardi, N., Hogan, M. J., Porter, F. W., & Weissman, D. (2018). mRNA vaccines—A new era in vaccinology. *Nature Reviews. Drug Discovery, 174*(17), 261–279 2018.

Parodi, A., Corbo, C., Cevenini, A., Molinaro, R., Palomba, R., Pandolfi, L., ... Tasciotti, E. (2015). Enabling cytoplasmic delivery and organelle targeting by surface modification of nanocarriers. *Nanomedicine: Nanotechnology, Biology, and Medicine, 10*, 1923.

Pastor, F., Berraondo, P., Etxeberria, I., Frederick, J., Sahin, U., Gilboa, E., & Melero, I. (2018). An RNA toolbox for cancer immunotherapy. *Nature Reviews. Drug Discovery, 1710*(17), 751–767.

Petros, R. A., & Desimone, J. M. (2010). Strategies in the design of nanoparticles for therapeutic applications. *Nature Reviews. Drug Discovery, 9*, 615–627.

Phan, G. Q., & Rosenberg, S. A. (2013). Adoptive cell transfer for patients with metastatic melanoma: The potential and promise of cancer immunotherapy. *Cancer Control: Journal of the Moffitt Cancer Center, 20*, 289–297.

Qi, C., Musetti, S., Fu, L. H., Zhu, Y. J., & Huang, L. (2019). Biomolecule-assisted green synthesis of nanostructured calcium phosphates and their biomedical applications. *Chemical Society Reviews, 48*, 2698–2737.

Rosenblum, D., Gutkin, A., Kedmi, R., Ramishetti, S., Veiga, N., Jacobi, A. M., ... Peer, D. (2020). CRISPR–Cas9 genome editing using targeted lipid nanoparticles for cancer therapy. *Science Advances, 6*, 9450–9468.

Rosewell Shaw, A., Porter, C. E., Watanabe, N., Tanoue, K., Sikora, A., Gottschalk, S., ... Suzuki, M. (2017). Adenovirotherapy delivering cytokine and checkpoint inhibitor augments CAR T cells against metastatic head and neck cancer. *Molecular Therapy: The Journal of the American Society of Gene Therapy, 25*, 2440–2451.

Ruoslahti, E. (2012). Peptides as targeting elements and tissue penetration devices for nanoparticles. *Advanced Materials, 24*, 3747–3756.

Sahin, U., Karikó, K., & Türeci, Ö. (2014). mRNA-based therapeutics—Developing a new class of drugs. *Nature Reviews. Drug Discovery, 1310*(13), 759–780.

Sandra, F., Khaliq, N. U., Sunna, A., & Care, A. (2019). Developing protein-based nanoparticles as versatile delivery systems for cancer therapy and imaging. *Nanomater, 9,* 1329.

Santos, S. A., Vidigal, P. M. P., Thrimawithana, A., Betancourth, B. M. L., Guimarães, L. M. S., Templeton, M. D., & Alfenas, A. C. (2020). Comparative genomic and transcriptomic analyses reveal different pathogenicity-related genes among three eucalyptus fungal pathogens. *Fungal Genetics and Biology: FG & B, 137,* 103332.

Scott, C. C., Vacca, F., & Gruenberg, J. (2014). Endosome maturation, transport and functions. *Seminars in Cell & Developmental Biology, 31,* 2–10.

Sebastian, M., Papachristofilou, A., Weiss, C., Früh, M., Cathomas, R., Hilbe, W., ... Zippelius, A. (2014). Phase Ib study evaluating a self-adjuvanted mRNA cancer vaccine (RNActive®) combined with local radiation as consolidation and maintenance treatment for patients with stage IV non-small cell lung cancer. *BMC Cancer, 14.*

Seyhan, A. A. (2019). Lost in translation: The valley of death across preclinical and clinical divide – identification of problems and overcoming obstacles. *Translational Medicine Communications, 41*(4), 1–19.

Shirley, J. L., de Jong, Y. P., Terhorst, C., & Herzog, R. W. (2020). Immune responses to viral gene therapy vectors. *Molecular Therapy: The Journal of the American Society of Gene Therapy, 28,* 709–722.

Singh, A., Qin, H., Fernandez, I., Wei, J., Lin, J., Kwak, L. W., & Roy, K. (2011). An injectable synthetic immune-priming center mediates efficient T-cell class switching and T-helper 1 response against B cell lymphoma. *Journal of Controlled Release: Official Journal of the Controlled Release Society, 155,* 184–192.

Song, W., Shen, L., Wang, Y., Liu, Q., Goodwin, T. J., Li, J., ... Huang, L. (2018). Synergistic and low adverse effect cancer immunotherapy by immunogenic chemotherapy and locally expressed PD-L1 trap. *Nature Communications, 91*(9), 1–11.

Sridharan, K., & Gogtay, N. J. (2016). Therapeutic nucleic acids: Current clinical status. *British Journal of Clinical Pharmacology, 82,* 659–672.

Stewart, M. P., Sharei, A., Ding, X., Sahay, G., Langer, R., & Jensen, K. F. (2016). In vitro and ex vivo strategies for intracellular delivery. *Nature, 5387624*(538), 183–192.

Verbeke, C. S., Gordo, S., Schubert, D. A., Lewin, S. A., Desai, R. M., Dobbins, J., ... Mooney, D. J. (2017). Multicomponent injectable hydrogels for antigen-specific tolerogenic immune modulation. *Advanced Healthcare Materials, 6.*

Verbeke, C. S., & Mooney, D. J. (2015). Injectable, pore-forming hydrogels for in vivo enrichment of immature dendritic cells. *Advanced Healthcare Materials, 4,* 2677–2687.

Verma, I. M., & Somia, N. (1997). Gene therapy—Promises, problems and prospects. *Nature, 389(6648),* 239–242.

Vollmer, J., & Krieg, A. M. (2009). Immunotherapeutic applications of CpG oligodeoxynucleotide TLR9 agonists. *Advanced Drug Delivery Reviews, 61,* 195–204.

Walsh, C. L., Nguyen, J., Tiffany, M. R., & Szoka, F. C. (2013). Synthesis, characterization, and evaluation of ionizable lysine-based lipids for siRNA delivery. *Bioconjugate Chemistry, 24,* 36–43.

Wang, J., Hu, Y., & Huang, H. (2017). Acute lymphoblastic leukemia relapse after CD19-targeted chimeric antigen receptor T cell therapy. *Journal of Leukocyte Biology, 102,* 1347–1356.

Wang, Z., Day, N., Trifillis, P., & Kiledjian, M. (1999). An mRNA stability complex functions with poly(A)-binding protein to stabilize mRNA in vitro. *Molecular and Cellular Biology, 19,* 4552–4560.

Whitehead, K. A., Langer, R., & Anderson, D. G. (2009). Knocking down barriers: Advances in siRNA delivery. *Nature Reviews. Drug Discovery, 82*(8), 129–138.

Xie, N., Shen, G., Gao, W., Huang, Z., Huang, C., & Fu, L. (2023). Neoantigens: Promising targets for cancer therapy. *Signal Transduction and Targeted Therapy, 81*(8), 1–38 2022.

Xu, Z., & Moyle, P. M. (2018). Bioconjugation approaches to producing subunit vaccines composed of protein or peptide antigens and covalently attached toll-like receptor ligands. *Bioconjugate Chemistry, 29*, 572–586.

Yin, H., Kanasty, R. L., Eltoukhy, A. A., Vegas, A. J., Dorkin, J. R., & Anderson, D. G. (2014). Non-viral vectors for gene-based therapy. *Nature Reviews. Genetics, 158*(15), 541–555.

Yin, H., Kauffman, K. J., & Anderson, D. G. (2017). Delivery technologies for genome editing. *Nature Reviews. Drug Discovery, 16*, 387–399.

Zámečník, J., Vargová, L., Homola, A., Kodet, R., & Syková, Es (2004). Extracellular matrix glycoproteins and diffusion barriers in human astrocytic tumours. *Neuropathology and Applied Neurobiology, 30*, 338–350.

Zelphati, O., & Szoka, F. C. (1996). Mechanism of oligonucleotide release from cationic liposomes. *Proceedings of the National Academy of Sciences of the United States of America, 93*, 11493–11498.

Ziller, A., Nogueira, S. S., Hühn, E., Funari, S. S., Brezesinski, G., Hartmann, H., ... Langguth, P. (2018). Incorporation of mRNA in lamellar lipid matrices for parenteral administration. *Molecular Pharmaceutics, 15*, 642–651.

CHAPTER THREE

Plasmid DNA and mRNA delivery: Approaches and challenges

Arun Kumar Singh[a],*, Karan Goel[b] ⓘ, and Meenakshi Dhanawat[c] ⓘ

[a]Department of Pharmacy, Vivekananda Global University, Jaipur, Rajasthan, India
[b]M.M College of Pharmacy, Maharishi Markandeshwar (Deemed to be University), Mullana–Ambala, Haryana, India
[c]Amity Institute of Pharmacy, Amity University Haryana, Amity Education Valley, Panchgaon, Manesar, Gurugram, Haryana, India
*Corresponding author. e-mail address: Arunthakur01996@gmail.com

Contents

Abstract

for delivery of plasmid DNA and mRNA transform biology and medicine, offering powerful tools for gene therapy, vaccine development, cancer immunotherapy, and regenerative medicine. Plasmid DNA provides a relatively stable and sustained expression of the genes which also provides the basic groundwork for long-lasting therapeutic. At the same time, mRNA has also demonstrated more appropriateness for dynamic and time-sensitive applications due to its short-lived and accurate translation capabilities, such as during the development of mRNA-based COVID-19 vaccines. Despite their unique advantages, however, the efficient delivery of these biomolecules poses challenges including immune system activation, enzymatic

Advances in Immunology, Volume 165
ISSN 0065-2776, https://doi.org/10.1016/bs.ai.2024.12.001

degradation, and limited cellular uptake. The structural and functional features of plasmid DNA and mRNA highlighted the positive functions that underpin their complementary roles in next-generation biomedical applications. In addition, it highlights the novel delivery routes across lipid nanoparticles, polymeric systems, biomimetic carriers, and hybrid applied sciences which can resolve long-standing challenges to efficient distribution. Emerging technologies such as CRISPR gene editing, self-amplifying RNA, and multiplexed nanoparticles are also increasing the utility of these systems. Significant advances in the delivery of plasmid DNA and mRNA molecules have revolutionized vaccine development, opened new avenues in personalized medicine, and have also inspired a future with engineerable tissues. As these innovations develop, they are predicted to go beyond current limitations and bring around a fresh era of accurate medication taking on one of the global healthcare's most complex challenges. Our revolutionary delivery methods provide stability and simplicity, transforming medical advances.

1. Introduction

Generative medicine, vaccine research, and plasmid DNA/mRNA delivery have all seen dramatic advancements in recent years (Uchida, 2022). Continual gene editing and expression are made possible by circular, double-stranded plasmid DNA. Its use in DNA vaccines, recombinant protein production, and gene cloning stems from its ability to replicate autonomously inside host cells ("905. Characterization of Plasmid DNA/ mRNA Co-Delivery In Vitro," 2008; Ahlemeyer, Colasante, & Baumgart-Vogt, 2020). Rapid and controlled expression of therapeutic proteins or antigens is made possible by messenger RNA (mRNA), a single-stranded molecule that acts as a transient intermediate in protein synthesis, in contrast to host DNA. The COVID-19 vaccine demonstrates that messenger RNA's direct protein synthesis makes it ideal for uses requiring rapid and precise therapeutic results. Plasmid DNA and messenger RNA work well together, but for therapeutic purposes, accurate and efficient distribution is crucial. Intrinsic barriers to children, such as immune system activation, enzymatic degradation, and cellular uptake, must be complex solutions. Advances in nanotechnology, chemical modification, and hybrid systems have increased the stability, specificity, and efficiency of many delivery systems and solved some of the problems (Martínez, Lampaya, Larraga, Magallón, & Casabona, 2023). Properties and functions of plasmid DNA and mRNA, their place in advanced biomedical research, and the various physical, chemical, and biological applications developed for their control. Explores the clinical applications of these biomolecules and highlights their potential in personalized medicine, immunotherapy, and regenerative medicine. By overcoming barriers and utilizing the unique properties of plasmid DNA and mRNA, this technology will revolutionize modern medicine and biotechnology (Aoyama, Kimura, Matsui, & Nozawa, 2023).

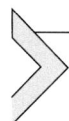

2. Overview of plasmid DNA and mRNA: structure and function

Two basic macromolecules in molecular biology are plasmid DNA and mRNA. Their structure and function lead them to find special biotechnological uses. Circular, bidirectional DNA found in plasmids might be one to two hundred kilobase pairs. Especially remarkable is their capacity for autonomous proliferation from an origin of replication (Clark & Pazdernik, 2013). Especially in bacteria but also in certain eukaryotes, plasmids may remain stable and replicate independently within host cells. To aid in identifying transformed cells, cloned plasmids have multiple closure sites (MCS) for invading DNA fragments and selectable indicators such as an antibiotic resistance gene. Promoter sequences such as T7 or CMV may actively transcribe other helpful biomolecules, medicinal proteins, and enzymes (Garg & Sandhir, 1999; Laroui, Sitaraman, & Merlin, 2012). Because they transfer antibiotic resistance, toxin generation, or microbial variety genes, plasmids are fundamental for bacterial adaptation. Since plasmids may express certain features, they have both scientific and medicinal applications. Scientists have developed gene therapy, DNA vaccines, recombinant protein synthesis, and gene amplification using the tools (Tolmasky, 2013).

Molecular biology is built around a linear, single-stranded molecule known as messenger RNA (mRNA). Generated as a complementary strand to template DNA during transcription and altered post-transcriptionally to provide better stability and support translation, mRNA is schematically Messenger RNA that binds to the ribosome using its methylguanosine 5′ cap. Ultimately, the amino acid sequence of a protein follows CDS. As CDS flanking regions, UTRs control stability and translation efficiency. At last, a 3′ poly(A) tail stabilizes and helps translocation (Tolmasky, 2013). Messenger RNA (mRNA) is perfect for transitory protein synthesis unlike plasmid DNA as it degrades quickly after translation. mRNA-based vaccinations show how dynamically biomedical technology is developing. Strong adaptive immune responses are produced by immunogenic proteins such as the SARS-CoV-2 spike protein found in such vaccinations. Messenger RNA (mRNA) in gene therapy generates therapeutic proteins momentarily without altering host genetic material. Transcriptomic research uses gene expression patterns to detect and define both healthy and diseased states (James & Robert, 1996; Travisano, 2001).

Though mass-produced using similar techniques, plasmid DNA and messenger RNA have functionally different uses. Because they may be stable and genetically altered, plasmids are crucial in both gene therapy and recombinant protein production. mRNA's ephemerality and direct access to protein synthesis, however, make it perfect for dynamic sitting and temporary uses such as vaccinations and medications requiring precisely regulated temporal expression. These biomolecules show how modern biotechnology is promoted by stability and transience complementing molecular biology (Gahtan, Olson, & Sumpio, 2002).

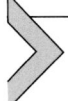

3. Significance of plasmid DNA and mRNA administration in biomedical research

Gene therapy, regenerative medicine, vaccine development, and other biomedical investigations rely on plasmid DNA and messenger RNA delivery. The effectiveness of both therapeutic and research outcomes relies on the precision with which biomolecules are administered, overturning context dependency for these biomolecules onto certain delivery mechanisms that determine their biological outcomes (Jahanafrooz et al., 2020; Martínez-Puente et al., 2022).

3.1 Plasmid DNA delivery

A plasmid containing DNA that encodes therapeutic proteins, vaccination antigens, regulatory RNA molecules, or stable carriers for long-term gene expression. Delivery is essential to gene therapy a treatment that corrects genetic issues by using plasmid DNA carrying functional copies of defective genes (Teo, Cheng, Hedrick, & Yang, 2016). In addition, DNA vaccines express genes that encode antigens to induce potent immunogenic immune responses using plasmid DNA. However, the main challenge is to over-come cellular barriers to delivery i.e. getting across the plasma membrane, escaping from endosomal degradation, and ensuring entry to the nucleus for transcription. One process of delivery is viral vectors, such as adenoviruses and lentiviruses (Hirko, Tang, & Hughes, 2003). However, vectors that are highly competent at doing this can lead to immunogenicity and insertional mutagenesis. Lipid nanoparticles (LNPs), electroporation, and polymeric nanoparticles are non-viral approaches that ensure safety. These approaches are improving and focusing on biomaterial engineering and nanotechnology (Hirko et al., 2003; Martínez-Puente et al., 2022; Song et al., 2017).

3.2 mRNA delivery

Due to its transitory and non-integrative nature, mRNA serves as an effective alternative to DNA for applications necessitating temporary protein production, including cancer immunotherapies and vaccinations. Messenger RNA does not require nuclear entry as plasmid DNA, allowing direct cytoplasmic translation (Jahanafrooz et al., 2020). This reduces the chance of mutagenesis and increases the probability of therapeutic effect. This fragile molecule needs to be delivered elegantly, geared up for the perfect cellular uptake, and without getting decomposed by enzymes, which mRNA is naturally sensitive to (Islam et al., 2015; Wadhwa, Aljabbari, Lokras, Foged, & Thakur, 2020). The Pfizer-BioNTech and Moderna COVID-19 vaccines demonstrated lipid nanoparticles as gold standard vectors for mRNA delivery. The messenger RNA (mRNA) is encapsulated in these nucleoprotein nanoparticles to protect mRNA from degradation by nucleases and allow uptake of cellular endocytosis (Islam et al., 2015; Qin, Du, & Sun, 2021; Wadhwa et al., 2020).

3.3 Significance in biomedical research

Plasmid and messenger RNA delivery is foundational to several fields of study, one of which is personalized medicine, which uses patients' genetic information to create unique treatment plans. One example is cancer immunotherapy, which uses messenger RNA (mRNA) vaccines to teach the immune system to recognize and destroy cancer cells (Islam et al., 2015). Novel CAR T-cell therapies have been developed using plasmid DNA. To combat cancer, these medicines modify immune cells. Vaccines for new infectious illnesses, such as COVID-19, may now be produced more quickly because of the efficient synthesis and modification of mRNA (Xiao et al., 2022). Genome editing tools such as CRISPR-Cas9 provide light on gene regulation and function by modifying specific genes using plasmid DNA or messenger RNA. In addition, regenerative medicine makes use of plasmid DNA and messenger RNA to transform somatic cells into induced pluripotent stem cells (iPSCs), which opens up new avenues of study in developmental biology and the possibility of cell treatments tailored to individual patients (Chaudhary, Weissman, & Whitehead, 2021; Xiao et al., 2022). Distributing plasmid DNA and messenger RNA is crucial for gene and molecular therapy. Innovative delivery strategies such as hybrid systems, biodegradable polymers, tissue-targeting nanoparticles, and others are needed to address immunogenicity, off-target effects, and industrial scalability. Expanding scientific research and bringing break-through treatments to market may be aided by these outcomes (Chaudhary et al., 2021; Kubiatowicz, Mohapatra, Krishnan, Fang, & Zhang, 2022; Xiao et al., 2022).

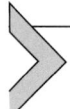

4. Key challenges in methods for delivering mRNA and plasmid DNA

Biomedicine still struggles to transport messenger RNA and plasmid DNA efficiently. Immune recognition and cellular absorption must be overcome to improve these systems' efficacy and safety (Liu, 2019).

4.1 Immune response

The immune system makes it hard for plasmid DNA and messenger RNA to spread. Because of the potential foreignness of biomolecules and their carriers, immunogenicity might occur. The presence of unmethylated CpG sequences, which are prevalent in bacterial DNA and activate TLR9, allows the innate immune system to recognize plasmid DNA (Abdulhaqq & Weiner, 2008; Donnelly, Wahren, & Liu, 2005). Therapeutic effec-tiveness and inflammation may be diminished by immune system activa-tion. The use of viral vectors to deliver plasmids has the potential to elicit strong immune responses and amplify side effects, which might make repeated dosage impractical. mRNA becomes immunogenic when pattern recognition receptors (PRRs) such as TLRs, RIG-I, and TLR7 are acti-vated. Intrasystemic inflammation and a short window of opportunity for treatment are consequences of unaltered messenger RNA. Modern developments in mRNA vaccine development, such as sequence optimi-zation and the use of chemically modified nucleotides (such as pseudour-idine), have mitigated these side effects. It is also possible for delivery vehicles, such as lipid nanoparticles (LNPs), to trigger complement-system hypersensitivity. The need for delivery methods that are immunologically inactive to decrease off-target immune activation is underscored by these responses, which are often moderate (Babiuk, 2003; Suschak, Williams, & Schmaljohn, 2017).

4.2 Cellular uptake

The lipid bilayer presents obstacles to the entry of messenger RNA (mRNA) and plasmid DNA into cells, resulting in difficulties in cellular absorption. The process of gene expression after plasmid DNA delivery is contingent upon nuclear localization and cellular absorption. Active distribution is necessary since passive diffusion is not an option due to the hydrophilicity and size of plasmid DNA. Security concerns and the difficulty of producing viral vectors restrict their use, even though they increase acceptability. While liposomes, electroporation, and polymeric nanoparticles may enhance cellular absorption, viral techniques are usually more successful when it comes to transfection. Since lysosomes often ensnare and destroy the plasmid DNA route to the nucleus, endosomal escape poses an additional obstacle (Kawakami, Higuchi, & Hashida, 2008; Spagnou, Miller, & Keller, 2004).

Moving from the nucleus to the cytoplasm is no picnic for messenger RNA, even if it doesn't need nuclear entrance. Its fragility and sensitivity to both extracellular and intracellular RNases make delivery more difficult. The encapsulation and protection provided by lipid nanoparticles make them very suitable for the endocytosis and cellular absorption of messenger RNA (mRNA). It may be more difficult for mRNA to avoid endosomal degradation in lysosomal compartments. Modern innovations, such as ionizable lipids in LNPs, have allowed endosome escape by destabilizing endosomal membranes. It is necessary to optimize certain cell types and tissues (Oh et al., 2002; Youn & Chung, 2015).

Improving methods of delivering plasmid DNA and messenger RNA requires addressing challenges related to immune response and cellular absorption. Delivery vehicles with improved endosomal escape, chemical modifications to reduce immunogenicity, and targeting of certain cell types or tissues are all necessary to overcome these challenges. If mRNA and plasmid DNA treatments could be made safer and more effective, they may become more popular in both the lab and the clinic (Denis-Mize et al., 2000; Scholz & Wagner, 2012; Uchida, 2022) and are showed in (Fig. 1).

Targeted Lipid Nanoparticles for Enhanced mRNA Delivery: Overcoming Cellular and Endosomal Barriers

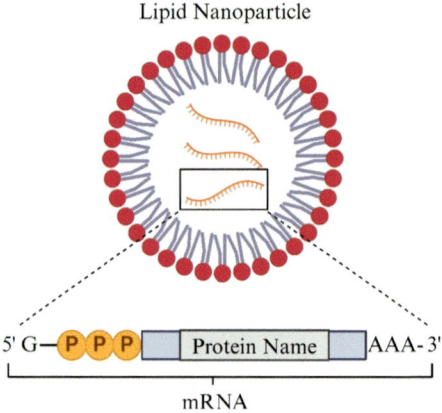

Fig. 1 Targeted lipid nanoparticles for enhanced mRNA delivery: overcoming cellular and endosomal barriers.

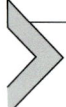

5. Physical techniques for the delivery of plasmid DNA and mRNA

Mechanical forces penetrate physiological barriers to directly transfer plasmid DNA and mRNA to target cells, giving great accuracy and utility in research and therapy (Uchida, 2022) and are mentioned in (Table 1).

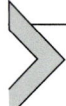

6. Chemical approaches for the delivery of plasmid DNA and mRNA

Chemical transfer of plasmid DNA and messenger RNA with little risk by use of specifically designed molecules. These approaches preserve DNA, improve cellular uptake, and narrow concentrated on specific organs and are referred in (Table 2).

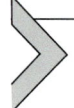

7. Biological techniques for the delivery of plasmid DNA and mRNA

The utilization of natural processes, often found in viruses or other cells, allows biological approaches to transfer plasmid DNA and messenger RNA

Table 1 Physical techniques for the delivery of plasmid DNA and mRNA.

Method	Mechanism	Applications	Advantages	Challenges	References
Electroporation	High-voltage electrical pulses create temporary pores in the cell membrane, enabling charged molecules like plasmid DNA or mRNA to enter cells via electrophoresis.	• Gene therapy (e.g., CAR-T cell engineering). Delivery of CRISPR–Cas9 components.Vaccine development using mRNA.	• High transfection efficiency, including in difficult-to-transfect cells.Compatible with a broad range of cell types.	• Can induce cell death due to excessive electrical pulses.Limited scalability for in vivo applications.	Young and Dean (2015)
Gene Gun	DNA or RNA-coated gold or tungsten particles are propelled into cells at high velocity using compressed gas, achieving intracellular delivery.	• DNA vaccination, particularly intradermal delivery. • Experimental use in tissue-specific mRNA delivery.	• Allows localized and targeted delivery.Effective in overcoming physical barriers in skin and plant cells.	• Tissue damage from high particle velocity.Limited efficiency for large-scale applications.	Jinturkar, Rathi, and Misra (2011)
Sonoporation	Ultrasound waves generate cavitation bubbles that collapse to create mechanical forces, temporarily disrupting the cell membrane for nucleic acid entry.	• Localized delivery of plasmid DNA in tumor-targeted gene therapy.Therapeutic mRNA delivery to liver and skeletal muscle.	• Non-invasive and ultrasound-guided for tissue specificity.Can be combined with other delivery methods for enhanced efficiency.	• Risk of cell and tissue damage from excessive cavitation.Requires precise control of ultrasound parameters for reproducibility and safety.	Shapiro et al. (2016)

Table 2 Chemical approaches for the delivery of plasmid DNA and mRNA.

Delivery system	Recent advances	Applications	Advantages	Challenges	References
Lipid-Based Systems	• Development of next-generation lipid nanoparticles (LNPs) with ionizable lipids for enhanced endosomal escape and reduced toxicity. • Functionalized LNPs for cell- or tissue-specific targeting (e.g., liver, immune cells).	• mRNA vaccines for infectious diseases (e.g., COVID−19). • CRISPR-Cas9 delivery for gene editing.	• High transfection efficiency. • Biodegradable and tunable.	• Potential immunogenicity of lipid components. • Stability during storage and transport remains challenging.	Maurer et al. (1999)
Polymer-Based Systems	• Design of biodegradable polymers like poly (beta-amino esters) for reduced cytotoxicity. • Use of zwitterionic polymers to improve stability in biological environments.	• Delivery of plasmid DNA in tissue engineering. • mRNA delivery for cancer immunotherapy.	• Customizable for specific tissues. • Controlled release profiles for sustained delivery.	• Variable transfection efficiency in different cell types. • Complex production processes.	Yang, Mixich, Boonstra, and Cabral (2023)
Hybrid Systems	• Combination of lipids and polymers (e.g., lipid-polymer hybrid	• Gene therapy for rare diseases.	• Synergistic benefits: improved	• Optimization of formulation complexity.	Seaberg et al. (2021)

	nanoparticles) to integrate the advantages of both systems. • Use of dendrimers and micelles for enhanced stability and cellular uptake.	• Delivery of therapeutic mRNA in regenerative medicine.	efficiency, biocompatibility, and targeting.	• Scalability issues for clinical-grade production.	
Biomimetic Systems	• Use of extracellular vesicles (e.g., exosomes) as natural carriers for DNA and RNA. • Cell membrane-coated nanoparticles for immune evasion and prolonged circulation.	• Therapeutic delivery for cancer and immune disorders.	• Biocompatible and low immunogenicity. • Exploit natural cellular uptake mechanisms.	• Limited production scalability. • Potential variability due to biological sourcing of vesicles.	Yin et al. (2024)
Charge-Adaptable Systems	• Development of pH-sensitive nanoparticles that change charge for better endosomal escape and cytoplasmic release. • Dynamic carriers that adjust charge density based on the cellular environment.	• Delivery of mRNA in vaccines and gene therapies.	• Enhanced specificity and reduced off-target effects.	• Requires precise tuning for optimal performance. • High cost of developing adaptable materials.	Liang, Huang, and Liu (2021)

into cells more effectively. These approaches are selective and compatible with cells; nonetheless, they need fine-tuning to minimize immunogenicity and toxicity (Guan & Rosenecker, 2017) and are mentioned in (Table 3).

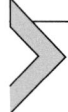

8. Cutting-edge methods for transporting mRNA and plasmid DNA

The development of safer, more efficient, and tailored methods has led to the advancement of plasmid DNA and mRNA delivery. By optimizing innovative delivery systems, nucleic acid preservation, off-target effects are reduced, and cellular absorption is enhanced and are showed in (Table 4).

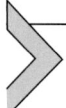

9. Clinical applications: plasmid DNA and mRNA delivery systems

The invention of many platforms for the treatment and prevention of diseases, made possible by DNA and mRNA delivery technologies, has revolutionized medicine. Vaccination methods, genetic editing, and transient production of medicinal proteins all rely on these systems. The therapeutic use of delivery technology has expanded across illnesses due to recent advancements and are mentioned in (Table 5).

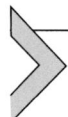

10. Regulatory challenges for therapeutic plasmid DNA and mRNA delivery

There has to be control over the quality, efficacy, and safety of plasmid DNA and mRNA-based therapies because of how quickly they are developing, particularly in light of the COVID-19 pandemic (Donnelly et al., 2005). Clinical trials, post-market monitoring, preclinical research, and manufacturing are all covered by these regulations. Compared to viral approaches, plasmid DNA and mRNA therapies are safer due to transient expression and non-integrative processes (Hardee et al., 2017; Seow & Wood, 2009). It is necessary to evaluate immunogenicity, off-target effects, and the efficacy of administration. Manufacturing standards are necessary for regulatory compliance. Good Manufacturing Practices are necessary to ensure the purity and consistency of plasmid DNA and messenger RNA batches. The problems of scalability and quality may be solved by using automated quality

Table 3 Biological techniques for the delivery of plasmid DNA and mRNA.

Method	Mechanism	Applications	Advantages	Challenges	References
Viral Vectors	Engineered viruses (e.g., lentivirus, adenovirus, AAV) are used to deliver genetic material into cells by exploiting their natural infection pathways.	• Gene therapy for inherited diseases. • Delivery of therapeutic mRNA and plasmid DNA.	• High transfection efficiency. • Long-term expression for DNA delivery.	• Immunogenicity and toxicity risks. • Expensive and complex production.	Hardee, Arévalo-Soliz, Hornstein, and Zechiedrich (2017)
Bacterial Vectors	Modified bacteria (e.g., *Salmonella, E. coli*) transport plasmid DNA into cells, often leveraging natural secretion systems like type III secretion systems (T3SS).	• Cancer immunotherapy. • Vaccine development using DNA or RNA.	• Targeted delivery to specific tissues. • Potential for intracellular persistence.	• Risk of systemic infection. • Limited efficiency compared to viral vectors.	Seow and Wood (2009)
Extracellular Vesicles	Natural carriers like exosomes are loaded with plasmid DNA or mRNA and delivered to target cells, exploiting their innate biocompatibility and cellular uptake mechanisms.	• Cancer therapeutics. • Delivery of regulatory RNA or mRNA for immune modulation.	• High biocompatibility. • Avoids immune recognition.	• Limited scalability for clinical use. • Potential variability in vesicle production.	Roerig and Schulz-Siegmund (2023)

(continued)

Table 3 Biological techniques for the delivery of plasmid DNA and mRNA. (*cont'd*)

Method	Mechanism	Applications	Advantages	Challenges	References
Protein–Based Carriers	Fusion proteins or peptide-based carriers bind plasmid DNA or mRNA, facilitating cellular uptake via receptor-mediated endocytosis or membrane fusion.	• Delivery of therapeutic mRNA for protein replacement therapies.	• Target-specific delivery via receptor targeting. • Low immunogenicity with engineered designs.	• High cost of synthesis. • Stability issues during production and delivery.	Uherek and Wels (2000)
Live-Cell Delivery	Direct delivery using living cells (e.g., T cells or macrophages) as "vehicles" to carry plasmid DNA or mRNA into target tissues through cell-cell interactions.	• CAR–T cell therapy (using plasmid DNA). • Immune modulation through mRNA delivery.	• Highly specific delivery. • Ability to home to specific tissues.	• Complex manufacturing process. • Potential immune rejection of the carrier cells.	Leonhardt et al. (2014)

Table 4 Cutting-edge methods for transporting mRNA and plasmid DNA.

Technology	Description	Applications	Advantages	Challenges	References
CRISPR-Assisted Delivery	Combines CRISPR–Cas systems with delivery vehicles (e.g., lipid nanoparticles or viral vectors) for precise genomic editing.	• Gene correction for genetic disorders. • Plasmid DNA delivery for gene editing applications.	• High specificity. • Programmable for targeted genome modifications.	• Delivery efficiency in vivo remains a challenge. • Risk of off-target effects.	Sundaresan et al. (2023)
Self-Amplifying RNA	mRNA is engineered to amplify itself within the cell, reducing the amount of material needed for delivery.	• mRNA vaccines for infectious diseases and cancer.	• Requires lower doses. Prolonged expression of the encoded protein.	• Potential for increased immunogenicity.	Omidi, Pourseif, Ansari, and Barar (2024)
DNA Origami-Based Delivery	Nucleic acids are folded into precise nanostructures that protect plasmid DNA or mRNA and enable targeted delivery.	• Precision delivery of genetic materials to specific cells.	• High biocompatibility. • Protects payloads from enzymatic degradation.	• Cost-intensive and technically challenging to produce at scale.	Zhang et al. (2018)
Microfluidic Delivery Platforms	Microfluidic devices are used to encapsulate plasmid DNA or mRNA into nanoparticles with precise control over size, charge, and surface properties.	• High-throughput development of nucleic acid therapies.	• Enhanced reproducibility. • Customizable for diverse applications.	• Requires specialized equipment.	Fardoost, Karimi, Govindaraju, Jamali, and Javanmard (2024)
Artificial Virus-Like Particles (VLPs)	Synthetic VLPs mimic viral vectors but are engineered to eliminate immunogenic components while retaining high efficiency.	• mRNA therapeutics for cardiovascular and metabolic diseases.	• Reduced immunogenicity compared to natural viral vectors. • High cellular uptake.	• Complex manufacturing and cost concerns.	Travassos, Martins, Fernandes, Correia, and Melo (2024)

(continued)

Table 4 Cutting-edge methods for transporting mRNA and plasmid DNA. (*cont'd*)

Technology	Description	Applications	Advantages	Challenges	References
pH–Responsive Carriers	Nanocarriers are engineered to change properties (e.g., charge or structure) in response to pH variations, enabling endosomal escape and cytoplasmic delivery.	• Targeted delivery for cancer therapy.	• Environment-responsive for controlled release. • Enhanced endosomal escape efficiency.	• Precise tuning of pH sensitivity is required.	Lu, Xing, Zheng, Huang, and Liang (2023)
Magnetofection	Uses magnetic fields to guide nanoparticle-bound plasmid DNA or mRNA to specific cells or tissues.	• Targeted delivery for regenerative medicine and localized therapies.	• High targeting precision. • Minimizes systemic exposure.	• Limited to superficial or accessible tissues.	Huang, Liu, Weng, and Chang (2021)
Hydrogel-Based Delivery	Incorporates plasmid DNA or mRNA into hydrogels for sustained and localized release.	• Wound healing. • Tissue engineering.	• Prolonged release and localized delivery. • Biocompatible and adaptable.	• Limited applications for systemic delivery.	Iqbal et al. (2023)

Table 5 Clinical applications: plasmid DNA and mRNA delivery systems.

Application area	Examples	Mechanism	Advantages	Challenges	References
Vaccines	• COVID–19 vaccines (e.g., Pfizer–BioNTech, Moderna mRNA vaccines). • Cancer vaccines targeting neoantigens.	Encodes antigens that stimulate an immune response.	• Rapid development and production. • Highly adaptable to emerging pathogens.	• Cold chain requirements for mRNA vaccines. • Potential for immune-related side effects.	Suschak et al. (2017)
Cancer Immunot-herapy	• CAR–T cell therapy using plasmid DNA. • mRNA vaccines for melanoma and lung cancer.	Modulates immune cells to recognize and destroy cancer cells.	• Personalized therapy for specific tumor antigens. • Non-integrative delivery avoids mutagenesis.	• High costs of production. • Need for robust delivery to immune cells.	Jahanafrooz et al. (2020), Miao, Zhang, and Huang (2021)
Genetic Disorders	• Treatment of hemophilia (e.g., factor IX expression via plasmid DNA). • Gene editing for sickle cell anemia using CRISPR–Cas9 with plasmid DNA.	Provides a template or editing tool for correcting genetic defects.	• Long-term therapeutic effects are possible with gene editing.	• Delivery to specific tissues remains a challenge.	Jit et al. (2022)

(continued)

Table 5 Clinical applications: plasmid DNA and mRNA delivery systems. (*cont'd*)

Application area	Examples	Mechanism	Advantages	Challenges	References
Infectious Diseases	• Zika virus mRNA vaccines. • Plasmid DNA vaccines for HPV-related cervical cancer.	Stimulates immune response to viral or bacterial antigens.	• Platform adaptability to various pathogens.	• Achieving long-lasting immunity.	Chaudhary et al. (2021)
Regenerative Medicine	• Delivery of growth factors for tissue repair (e.g., VEGF for angiogenesis via plasmid DNA).	Promotes cell proliferation and differentiation for tissue repair.	• Localized and transient expression minimizes off-target effects.	• Limited efficiency in complex tissues or organs.	Lorden, Levinson, and Leong (2015)
Neurological Disorders	• Delivery of neuroprotective factors (e.g., BDNF via mRNA) for treating neurodegenerative diseases.	Provides transient expression of therapeutic proteins in the CNS.	• Non-invasive options via lipid nanoparticles or intranasal delivery.	• Blood-brain barrier limits delivery efficiency.	Nguyen et al. (2024)
Cardiovascular Diseases	• Delivery of mRNA encoding VEGF for myocardial regeneration post-infarction.	Enhances vascular growth and repair in damaged cardiac tissue.	• Local delivery reduces systemic side effects.	• The short half-life of therapeutic proteins necessitates repeated dosing.	Rincon, Vanden Driessche, and Chuah (2015)
Rare Diseases	• Enzyme replacement therapy using plasmid DNA or mRNA for lysosomal storage disorders.	Provides transient expression of deficient enzymes.	• Potential for broader accessibility to rare disease patients.	• Requires tissue-specific targeting for efficacy.	Zhao, Hou, Vick, and Dong (2019)

control and continuous manufacturing (Martínez et al., 2023; Uchida, 2022). Lipid nanoparticles (LNPs) used as mRNA vaccines or therapeutic delivery systems should be thoroughly characterized, stabilized, and stored according to guidelines set forth by the FDA and EMA. When investigating biodistribution, toxicity, or immunogenicity, it is crucial to conduct preclinical safety studies. To reduce the need for animal testing and improve the accuracy of human response predictions, regulatory testing is making use of innovative in silico and organ-on-a-chip models. The design and risk–benefit ratio of clinical trials are meticulously examined by authorities. The pandemic's quick licensing of mRNA vaccines highlighted the need for adaptable regulatory frameworks and extensive safety testing (Omidi et al., 2024; Wadhwa et al., 2020).

The regulatory framework for delivery systems that combine biomimetic carriers with hybrid nanoparticles is a huge advance. Problems with regulation arise in systems that are complex (chemical, physical, and biological). Strong systems for identifying and assessing the safety of these technologies are necessary for clinical translation (Seaberg et al., 2021; Song et al., 2017). Approval is contingent upon clinical trial evidence of efficacy across diverse populations. To make sure drugs work for everyone, regulatory agencies put fair trial access and representation first. Conditional approval based on early findings and continued research has been established by the early approval of mRNA-based COVID-19 vaccines (Abdulhaqq & Weiner, 2008; Donnelly et al., 2005). Regulation is aided by post-market surveillance. Artificial intelligence (AI) and real-world data analytics are used by advanced pharmacovigilance systems to track adverse occurrences and long-term effects to enhance future medications (Furriel et al., 2024). New information gleaned from mRNA vaccines and other technological developments is hastening the transformation of plasmid DNA and mRNA treatment control. Innovative regulatory approaches and frameworks are allowing these revolutionary therapies to be accepted in healthcare systems across the globe despite challenges related to manufacturing, immunogenicity, and equitable access (Gopalakrishnan, Helmink, Spencer, Reuben, & Wargo, 2018; Li, You, Griffin, Feng, & Shan, 2018).

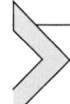

11. Emerging trends in innovative technologies and future strategies

New medical methods and technologies are hastening the spread of plasmid DNA and messenger RNA. A new development in nano-technology is the creation of multifunctional nanoparticles that can be used for the transport of adjuvants, plasmid DNA, and messenger RNA. These methods enhance cellular uptake and targeting while decreasing systemic toxicity. The new generation of ionizable lipid nanoparticles (LNPs) poses no danger when used therapeutically and breaks down naturally. There has been a recent uptick in the use of genetic and medical data to tailor delivery strategies (El-Kenawy et al., 2017; Kubiatowicz et al., 2022; Omidi et al., 2024). Precision medicine, which bases treatment decisions on patient-specific genetic markers and immune responses, may use this approach. High expenses and complexity of customization persist. To make them more accessible, researchers are working on transdermal patches, inhalable formulations, and intranasal devices. Our approaches allow for implementation with fewer resources while also improving patient adherence. With the help of AI, delivery system optimization is becoming better. To expedite research, AI algorithms may sift through massive information in search of optimal nanoparticle designs, formulations, and dosage regimens. The novel approach of self-amplifying mRNA (siRNA) raises therapeutic mRNA intracellularly, which reduces material requirements and improves efficacy. New clinical studies show promise for scalable vaccine production using SaRNA-based vaccines, which have the potential to elicit robust immune responses at low doses (Furriel et al., 2024; Scholz & Wagner, 2012; Spagnou et al., 2004).

Hybrid delivery methods are being expanded to include physical, biological, and chemical factors. Improved transfection and less off-target effects are achieved using nanoparticle-mediated electroporation. A significant intracellular delivery obstacle, endosomal entrapment, is being simultaneously addressed (Seaberg et al., 2021). Nucleic acid bioavailability to target cells may be enhanced by carriers that are both pH-sensitive and membrane-disruptive, allowing for better endosomal escape. The study of delivery involves overcoming biological obstacles, such as the blood-brain barrier. To combat neurological diseases like Parkinson's and Alzheimer's, researchers are creating engineered nanoparticles and receptor-mediated transport routes (Lu et al., 2023; Oh et al., 2002). Methods for delivering tissue-specific plasmid DNA and messenger RNA are being developed as part of regenerative medicine to repair damaged organs and mend wounds. Research into delivery vehicles for tissue engineering is focused on finding ways to both sustain and localize the expression of growth factors. Environmental stability improvements are necessary for mRNA and plasmid DNA treatments to overcome logistical hurdles in situations with limited resources. Reducing cold chain limits and enabling global distribution may be possible with formulations that have increased ambient temperature stability (Furriel et al., 2024).

The development of applications is being accelerated via the testing of universal technologies that can rapidly adapt to plasmid DNA and mRNA delivery. New biomaterials that respond to changes in pH and temperature are being created to provide targeted and accurate release. Plasmid DNA and messenger RNA are made more stable, useful, and therapeutically effective by synthetic biology. Revolutionizing nucleic acid therapies are these emerging technologies. As scientists find solutions to problems and refine delivery systems, plasmid DNA and messenger RNA technologies will transform regenerative treatments, personalized medicine, and global health (Uherek & Wels, 2000; Zhang et al., 2018).

12. Conclusion

Numerous ground-breaking therapies and discoveries have been made possible by the revolutionary nature of plasmid DNA and messenger RNA transport in molecular biology, biotechnology, and medicine. When it comes to temporary and precisely regulated protein synthesis, messenger RNA is superior to plasmid DNA, which is better for long-term genetic alteration and continuous protein expression (Donnelly et al., 2005; Song et al., 2017). Gene therapy, cancer immunotherapy, vaccine development, and regenerative medicine all rely on their synergistic qualities. These biomolecules can only be used with efficient delivery mechanisms that can withstand cellular absorption, enzymatic breakdown, and immunological activation (Gopalakrishnan et al., 2018; Li et al., 2018). Innovations in nanotechnology, biomaterials, and hybrid delivery systems have substantially improved efficacy, specificity, and safety in recent years. Lipidomic nanoparticles, polymer-based systems, and biomimetic carriers all work together to enhance targeted distribution and therapeutic benefits. In the future, these systems will be much better because of the incorporation of CRISPR-assisted delivery, pH-responsive carriers, and self-amplifying RNA (Scholz & Wagner, 2012; Spagnou et al., 2004). These initiatives aim to resolve concerns with scalability, stability, and tissue selectivity in mRNA and plasmid DNA-based therapeutics. New methods of delivering plasmid DNA and messenger RNA are revolutionizing healthcare and changing the face of medicine. Thanks to ongoing innovation and cross-disciplinary cooperation, these technologies have the potential to speed up personalized medicine, global health efforts, and regenerative therapies, all of which have the potential to improve patient outcomes on a global scale (Abdulhaqq & Weiner, 2008; Song et al., 2017).

References

Abdulhaqq, S. A., & Weiner, D. B. (2008). DNA vaccines: Developing new strategies to enhance immune responses. *Immunologic Research, 42*, 219. https://doi.org/10.1007/s12026-008-8076-3.

Ahlemeyer, B., Colasante, C., & Baumgart-Vogt, E. (2020). Analysis of the level of plasmid-derived mRNA in the presence of residual plasmid DNA by two-step quantitative RT-PCR. *Methods and Protocols, 3*, 40. https://doi.org/10.3390/mps3020040.

Aoyama, N., Kimura, S., Matsui, T., & Nozawa, T. (2023). In vivo tracking of plasmid DNA/mRNA: A novel labelling precursor for 89Zr positron emission tomography. *Bioorganic & Medicinal Chemistry Letters, 90*, 129332. https://doi.org/10.1016/j.bmcl.2023.129332.

Babiuk, L. (2003). Induction of immune responses by DNA vaccines in large animals. *Vaccine, 21*, 649–658. https://doi.org/10.1016/S0264-410X(02)00574-1.

Characterization of Plasmid DNA/mRNA Co-Delivery In Vitro. (2008). *Molecular Therapy, 16*, S337. https://doi.org/10.1016/S1525-0016(16)40308-4.

Chaudhary, N., Weissman, D., & Whitehead, K. A. (2021). mRNA vaccines for infectious diseases: Principles, delivery and clinical translation. *Nature Reviews. Drug Discovery, 20*, 817–838. https://doi.org/10.1038/s41573-021-00283-5.

Clark, D. P., & Pazdernik, N. J. (2013). *Plasmids. Molecular biology.* Elsevier, e473–e478. https://doi.org/10.1016/B978-0-12-378594-7.00055-X.

Denis-Mize, K. S., Dupuis, M., MacKichan, M. L., Singh, M., Doe, B., O'Hagan, D., ... Ott, G. (2000). Plasmid DNA adsorbed onto cationic microparticles mediates target gene expression and antigen presentation by dendritic cells. *Gene Therapy, 7*, 2105–2112. https://doi.org/10.1038/sj.gt.3301347.

Donnelly, J. J., Wahren, B., & Liu, M. A. (2005). DNA vaccines: Progress and challenges. *The Journal of Immunology, 175*, 633–639. https://doi.org/10.4049/jimmunol.175.2.633.

El-Kenawy, A. E.-M., Constantin, C., Hassan, S. M. A., Mostafa, A. M., Neves, A. F., De Araújo, T. G., & Neagu, M. (2017). *Nanomedicine in melanoma: Current trends and future perspectives. Cutaneous melanoma: Etiology and therapy.* Codon Publications, 143–159. https://doi.org/10.15586/codon.cutaneousmelanoma.2017.ch10.

Fardoost, A., Karimi, K., Govindaraju, H., Jamali, P., & Javanmard, M. (2024). Applications of microfluidics in mRNA vaccine development: A review. *Biomicrofluidics, 18*. https://doi.org/10.1063/5.0228447.

Furriel, B. C. R. S., Oliveira, B. D., Prôa, R., Paiva, J. Q., Loureiro, R. M., Calixto, W. P., ... Giavina-Bianchi, M. (2024). Artificial intelligence for skin cancer detection and classification for clinical environment: A systematic review. *Frontiers in Medicine (Lausanne), 10*. https://doi.org/10.3389/fmed.2023.1305954.

Gahtan, V., Olson, E. T., & Sumpio, B. E. (2002). Molecular biology: A brief overview. *Journal of Vascular Surgery: Official Publication, the Society for Vascular Surgery [and] International Society for Cardiovascular Surgery, North American Chapter, 35*, 563–568. https://doi.org/10.1067/mva.2002.120039.

Garg, S. K., & Sandhir, R. (1999). *Genetics of microorganisms | Bacteria. Encyclopedia of food microbiology.* Elsevier, 929–940. https://doi.org/10.1006/rwfm.1999.0740.

Gopalakrishnan, V., Helmink, B. A., Spencer, C. N., Reuben, A., & Wargo, J. A. (2018). The Influence of the gut microbiome on cancer, immunity, and cancer immunotherapy. *Cancer Cell, 33*, 570–580. https://doi.org/10.1016/j.ccell.2018.03.015.

Guan, S., & Rosenecker, J. (2017). Nanotechnologies in delivery of mRNA therapeutics using nonviral vector-based delivery systems. *Gene Therapy, 24*, 133–143. https://doi.org/10.1038/gt.2017.5.

Hardee, C., Arévalo-Soliz, L., Hornstein, B., & Zechiedrich, L. (2017). Advances in nonviral DNA vectors for gene therapy. *Genes (Basel), 8*, 65. https://doi.org/10.3390/genes8020065.

Hirko, A., Tang, F., & Hughes, J. (2003). Cationic lipid vectors for plasmid DNA delivery. *Current Medicinal Chemistry, 10*, 1185–1193. https://doi.org/10.2174/0929867033457412.

Huang, R.-Y., Liu, Z.-H., Weng, W.-H., & Chang, C.-W. (2021). Magnetic nanocomplexes for gene delivery applications. *Journal of Materials Chemistry B, 9*, 4267–4286. https://doi.org/10.1039/D0TB02713H.

Iqbal, Z., Rehman, K., Xia, J., Shabbir, M., Zaman, M., Liang, Y., & Duan, L. (2023). Biomaterial-assisted targeted and controlled delivery of CRISPR/Cas9 for precise gene editing. *Biomaterials Science, 11*, 3762–3783. https://doi.org/10.1039/D2BM01636B.

Islam, M. A., Reesor, E. K. G., Xu, Y., Zope, H. R., Zetter, B. R., & Shi, J. (2015). Biomaterials for mRNA delivery. *Biomaterials Science, 3*, 1519–1533. https://doi.org/10.1039/C5BM00198F.

Jahanafrooz, Z., Baradaran, B., Mosafer, J., Hashemzaei, M., Rezaei, T., Mokhtarzadeh, A., & Hamblin, M. R. (2020). Comparison of DNA and mRNA vaccines against cancer. *Drug Discovery Today, 25*, 552–560. https://doi.org/10.1016/j.drudis.2019.12.003.

James, D. B., & Robert, R. S. (1996). *Comparison of retention and expression of recombinant plasmids between suspended and biofilm-Bound bacteria degrading TCE*, 239–248. https://doi.org/10.1016/S0921-0423(96)80033-5.

Jinturkar, K. A., Rathi, M. N., & Misra, A. (2011). *Gene delivery using physical methods. Challenges in delivery of therapeutic genomics and proteomics*. Elsevier, 83–126. https://doi.org/10.1016/B978-0-12-384964-9.00003-7.

Jit, B. P., Pattnaik, S., Arya, R., Dash, R., Sahoo, S. S., Pradhan, B., ... Behera, R. K. (2022). Phytochemicals: A potential next generation agent for radioprotection. *Phytomedicine: International Journal of Phytotherapy and Phytopharmacology, 106*, 154188. https://doi.org/10.1016/j.phymed.2022.154188.

Kawakami, S., Higuchi, Y., & Hashida, M. (2008). Nonviral approaches for targeted delivery of plasmid DNA and oligonucleotide. *Journal of Pharmaceutical Sciences, 97*, 726–745. https://doi.org/10.1002/jps.21024.

Kubiatowicz, L. J., Mohapatra, A., Krishnan, N., Fang, R. H., & Zhang, L. (2022). mRNA nanomedicine: Design and recent applications. *Exploration, 2*. https://doi.org/10.1002/EXP.20210217.

Laroui, H., Sitaraman, S. V., & Merlin, D. (2012). *Gastrointestinal Delivery of Anti-inflammatory Nanoparticles*, 101–125. https://doi.org/10.1016/B978-0-12-391858-1.00006-X.

Leonhardt, C., Schwake, G., Stögbauer, T. R., Rappl, S., Kuhr, J.-T., Ligon, T. S., & Rädler, J. O. (2014). Single-cell mRNA transfection studies: Delivery, kinetics and statistics by numbers. *Nanomedicine: Nanotechnology, Biology, and Medicine, 10*, 679–688. https://doi.org/10.1016/j.nano.2013.11.008.

Li, Z., You, Y., Griffin, N., Feng, J., & Shan, F. (2018). Low-dose naltrexone (LDN): A promising treatment in immune-related diseases and cancer therapy. *International Immunopharmacology, 61*, 178–184. https://doi.org/10.1016/j.intimp.2018.05.020.

Liang, Y., Huang, L., & Liu, T. (2021). Development and delivery systems of mRNA vaccines. *Frontiers in Bioengineering and Biotechnology, 9*. https://doi.org/10.3389/fbioe.2021.718753.

Liu, M. A. (2019). A comparison of plasmid DNA and mRNA as vaccine technologies. *Vaccines (Basel), 7*, 37. https://doi.org/10.3390/vaccines7020037.

Lorden, E. R., Levinson, H. M., & Leong, K. W. (2015). Integration of drug, protein, and gene delivery systems with regenerative medicine. *Drug Delivery and Translational Research, 5*, 168–186. https://doi.org/10.1007/s13346-013-0165-8.

Lu, M., Xing, H., Zheng, A., Huang, Y., & Liang, X.-J. (2023). Overcoming pharmaceutical bottlenecks for nucleic acid drug development. *Accounts of Chemical Research, 56*, 224–236. https://doi.org/10.1021/acs.accounts.2c00464.

Martínez, J., Lampaya, V., Larraga, A., Magallón, H., & Casabona, D. (2023). Purification of linearized template plasmid DNA decreases double-stranded RNA formation during IVT reaction. *Frontiers in Molecular Biosciences, 10*. https://doi.org/10.3389/fmolb.2023. 1248511.

Martínez-Puente, D. H., Pérez-Trujillo, J. J., Zavala-Flores, L. M., García-García, A., Villanueva-Olivo, A., Rodríguez-Rocha, H., ... de, J. (2022). Plasmid DNA for therapeutic applications in cancer. *Pharmaceutics, 14*, 1861. https://doi.org/10.3390/ pharmaceutics14091861.

Maurer, N., Mori, A., Palmer, L., Monck, M. A., Mok, K. W. C., Mui, B., ... Cullis, P. R. (1999). Lipid-based systems for the intracellular delivery of genetic drugs. *Molecular Membrane Biology, 16*, 129–140. https://doi.org/10.1080/096876899294869.

Miao, L., Zhang, Y., & Huang, L. (2021). mRNA vaccine for cancer immunotherapy. *Molecular Cancer, 20*, 41. https://doi.org/10.1186/s12943-021-01335-5.

Nguyen, N. H., Nguyen-Thi, P., Nguyen, T. T., Bui, V. K. H., Nguyen, N. T. T., & Vo, G. V. (2024). Applications and developments of gene therapy drug delivery systems for neurological disorders. *Advances in Therapy (Weinh)*. https://doi.org/10.1002/adtp.202400269.

Oh, Y.-K., Suh, D., Kim, J. M., Choi, H.-G., Shin, K., & Ko, J. J. (2002). Polyethylenimine-mediated cellular uptake, nucleus trafficking and expression of cytokine plasmid DNA. *Gene Therapy, 9*, 1627–1632. https://doi.org/10.1038/sj.gt. 3301735.

Omidi, Y., Pourseif, M. M., Ansari, R. A., & Barar, J. (2024). Design and development of mRNA and self-amplifying mRNA vaccine nanoformulations. *Nanomedicine*, 1–27. https://doi.org/10.1080/17435889.2024.2419815.

Qin, M., Du, G., & Sun, X. (2021). Recent advances in the noninvasive delivery of mRNA. *Accounts of Chemical Research, 54*, 4262–4271. https://doi.org/10.1021/acs. accounts.1c00493.

Rincon, M. Y., Vanden Driessche, T., & Chuah, M. K. (2015). Gene therapy for cardiovascular disease: Advances in vector development, targeting, and delivery for clinical translation. *Cardiovascular Research, 108*, 4–20. https://doi.org/10.1093/cvr/cvv205.

Roerig, J., & Schulz-Siegmund, M. (2023). Standardization approaches for extracellular vesicle loading with oligonucleotides and biologics. *Small (Weinheim an der Bergstrasse, Germany), 19*. https://doi.org/10.1002/smll.202301763.

Scholz, C., & Wagner, E. (2012). Therapeutic plasmid DNA versus siRNA delivery: Common and different tasks for synthetic carriers. *Journal of Controlled Release, 161*, 554–565. https://doi.org/10.1016/j.jconrel.2011.11.014.

Seaberg, J., Montazerian, H., Hossen, M. N., Bhattacharya, R., Khademhosseini, A., & Mukherjee, P. (2021). Hybrid nanosystems for biomedical applications. *ACS Nano, 15*, 2099–2142. https://doi.org/10.1021/acsnano.0c09382.

Seow, Y., & Wood, M. J. (2009). Biological gene delivery vehicles: Beyond viral vectors. *Molecular Therapy, 17*, 767–777. https://doi.org/10.1038/mt.2009.41.

Shapiro, G., Wong, A. W., Bez, M., Yang, F., Tam, S., Even, L., ... Gazit, D. (2016). Multiparameter evaluation of in vivo gene delivery using ultrasound-guided, microbubble-enhanced sonoporation. *Journal of Controlled Release, 223*, 157–164. https://doi. org/10.1016/j.jconrel.2015.12.001.

Song, H., Yu, M., Lu, Y., Gu, Z., Yang, Y., Zhang, M., … Yu, C. (2017). Plasmid DNA delivery: Nanotopography matters. *Journal of the American Chemical Society, 139*, 18247–18254. https://doi.org/10.1021/jacs.7b08974.

Spagnou, S., Miller, A. D., & Keller, M. (2004). Lipidic carriers of siRNA: Differences in the formulation, cellular uptake, and delivery with plasmid DNA. *Biochemistry, 43*, 13348–13356. https://doi.org/10.1021/bi048950a.

Sundaresan, Y., Yacoub, S., Kodati, B., Amankwa, C. E., Raola, A., & Zode, G. (2023). Therapeutic applications of CRISPR/Cas9 gene editing technology for the treatment of ocular diseases. *The FEBS Journal, 290*, 5248–5269. https://doi.org/10.1111/febs.16771.

Suschak, J. J., Williams, J. A., & Schmaljohn, C. S. (2017). Advancements in DNA vaccine vectors, non-mechanical delivery methods, and molecular adjuvants to increase immunogenicity. *Human Vaccines & Immunotherapeutics, 13*, 2837–2848. https://doi.org/10.1080/21645515.2017.1330236.

Teo, P. Y., Cheng, W., Hedrick, J. L., & Yang, Y. Y. (2016). Co-delivery of drugs and plasmid DNA for cancer therapy. *Advanced Drug Delivery Reviews, 98*, 41–63. https://doi.org/10.1016/j.addr.2015.10.014.

Tolmasky, M. E. (2013). *Plasmids. Brenner's encyclopedia of genetics*. Elsevier, 362–366. https://doi.org/10.1016/B978-0-12-374984-0.01174-8.

Travassos, R., Martins, S. A., Fernandes, A., Correia, J. D. G., & Melo, R. (2024). Tailored viral-like particles as drivers of medical breakthroughs. *International Journal of Molecular Sciences, 25*, 6699. https://doi.org/10.3390/ijms25126699.

Travisano, M. (2001). *Bacterial genetics. Encyclopedia of biodiversity*. Elsevier, 339–350. https://doi.org/10.1016/B0-12-226865-2/00024-9.

Uchida, S. (2022). Delivery systems of plasmid DNA and messenger RNA for advanced therapies. *Pharmaceutics, 14*, 810. https://doi.org/10.3390/pharmaceutics14040810.

Uherek, C., & Wels, W. (2000). DNA-carrier proteins for targeted gene delivery. *Advanced Drug Delivery Reviews, 44*, 153–166. https://doi.org/10.1016/S0169-409X(00)00092-2.

Wadhwa, A., Aljabbari, A., Lokras, A., Foged, C., & Thakur, A. (2020). Opportunities and challenges in the delivery of mRNA-based vaccines. *Pharmaceutics, 12*, 102. https://doi.org/10.3390/pharmaceutics12020102.

Xiao, Y., Tang, Z., Huang, X., Chen, W., Zhou, J., Liu, H., … Tao, W. (2022). Emerging mRNA technologies: Delivery strategies and biomedical applications. *Chemical Society Reviews, 51*, 3828–3845. https://doi.org/10.1039/D1CS00617G.

Yang, W., Mixich, L., Boonstra, E., & Cabral, H. (2023). Polymer-based mRNA delivery strategies for advanced therapies. *Advanced Healthcare Materials, 12*. https://doi.org/10.1002/adhm.202202688.

Yin, M., Sun, H., Li, Y., Zhang, J., Wang, J., Liang, Y., & Zhang, K. (2024). Delivery of mRNA using biomimetic vectors: Progress and challenges. *Small (Weinheim an der Bergstrasse, Germany), 20*. https://doi.org/10.1002/smll.202402715.

Youn, H., & Chung, J.-K. (2015). Modified mRNA as an alternative to plasmid DNA (pDNA) for transcript replacement and vaccination therapy. *Expert Opinion on Biological Therapy, 15*, 1337–1348. https://doi.org/10.1517/14712598.2015.1057563.

Young, J. L., & Dean, D. A. (2015). *Electroporation-Mediated Gene Delivery*, 49–88. https://doi.org/10.1016/bs.adgen.2014.10.003.

Zhang, Y., Tu, J., Wang, D., Zhu, H., Maity, S. K., Qu, X., … Zhang, H. (2018). Programmable and multifunctional DNA-based materials for biomedical applications. *Advanced Materials, 30*. https://doi.org/10.1002/adma.201703658.

Zhao, W., Hou, X., Vick, O. G., & Dong, Y. (2019). RNA delivery biomaterials for the treatment of genetic and rare diseases. *Biomaterials, 217*, 119291. https://doi.org/10.1016/j.biomaterials.2019.119291.

CHAPTER FOUR

Progress in modifying and delivering mRNA therapies for cancer immunotherapy

Karan Goel[a], Isha Chawla[a], Garima[a], Meenakshi Dhanawat[b,*], and Pramila Chaubey[c,*]

[a]M.M College of Pharmacy, Maharishi Markandeshwar (Deemed to be University), Mullana-Ambala, Haryana, India
[b]Amity Institute of Pharmacy, Amity University Haryana, Amity Education Valley, Panchgaon, Manesar, Gurugram, Haryana, India
[c]Department of Pharmaceutics, College of Pharmacy, Shaqra University, Shaqra, Kingdom of Saudi Arabia
*Corresponding authors. e-mail address: meenakshi.iitbhu@gmail.com; cpramil@su.edu.sa

Contents

Abstract

Advancements in mRNA-based therapeutics have greatly enhanced cancer immunotherapy by using the immune system to specifically target and eradicate cancer cells. There has been notable advancement in tailoring and administering mRNA to treat cancer. Codon optimization, chemical alterations, and sequence manipulation are complex design methodologies employed in the production of mRNA vaccines and treatments. The goal is to improve the ability of the chemicals to stimulate an immune response, increase their ability to be translated into practical applications, and boost their stability. Lipid nanoparticles (LNPs) are currently the most efficient

ISSN 0065-2776, https://doi.org/10.1016/bs.ai.2024.10.004

means of delivering mRNA because they can withstand degradation, enhance cellular uptake, and facilitate endosomal escape. Scientists are currently investigating the possibility of using alternate methods of delivering substances, including as exosomes, lipoplexes, and polymeric nanoparticles, to enhance the ability to target specific tissues and minimize unwanted negative consequences. In addition, recent clinical trials and preclinical investigations have demonstrated encouraging findings in terms of the advancement of strong anti-tumor immune responses, long-lasting tumor shrinkage, and enhanced patient outcomes. The remaining challenges involve optimizing the equilibrium between tolerance and immunological activation, addressing systemic toxicity, and expanding manufacturing techniques. The upcoming study seeks to improve the design and dissemination of mRNA, include it in combination drugs, and investigate its therapeutic uses outside cancer. The advancement in cancer treatment represents a change in the current approach, highlighting the significant impact of mRNA technology in revolutionizing immunotherapy and enabling tailored cancer treatments.

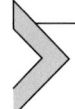

1. Introduction to mRNA therapies for cancer immunotherapy

mRNA therapies have emerged as a promising approach for cancer immunotherapy, with the potential to induce robust immune responses against tumor-specific antigens. Recent clinical trials have demonstrated encouraging results, with nearly 40 % of patients with stage IV melanoma showing vaccine-related clinical responses and generating T-cell responses against vaccine-encoded neoepitopes (Katopodi et al., 2024). In particular, using non-formulated mRNA vaccines containing tumor-associated antigens and dendritic cell-activating compounds has shown favorable clinical outcomes, highlighting the potential of mRNA therapies in cancer treatment.

The development of mRNA vaccines for cancer immunotherapy has been ongoing for decades, with significant progress in addressing challenges such as mRNA stability and in vivo delivery. Different types of mRNA vaccines, including replicating modified mRNA, unmodified mRNA, and virus-derived mRNA, have been developed to improve antigen expression and avoid gene integration (Duan, Wang, Zhang, Yang, & Zhang, 2022). Despite the challenges related to mRNA degradation and inefficient in vivo delivery, ongoing research and development efforts aim to overcome these limitations and further enhance the clinical application of mRNA vaccines in cancer immunotherapy (Pan, Fan, Han, Tong, & Guo, 2024).

2. Fundamentals of mRNA therapies

Messenger RNA (mRNA) treatments employ the body's cellular machinery to produce therapeutic proteins, a revolutionary medical paradigm. Membrane proteins are synthesized from single-stranded mRNA. Inherent mechanisms convert DNA into mRNA, which ribosomes translate into physiological proteins. Lab-made synthetic messenger RNA (mRNA) encodes enzyme, antigen, and hormone protein production in mRNA therapeutics. Lipid nanoparticles (LNPs) protect and aid mRNA absorption. Upon entrance, mRNA is translated into a therapeutic protein. Other treatments involve replacing a defective or malfunctioning protein, whereas microRNA (mRNA) vaccines induce an immunological response (Han, Noh et al., 2023; Kong, Kim, Kim, Suk, & Yang, 2023).

Immunizations, cancer treatments, and protein replacement employ mRNA therapy. The effectiveness of mRNA vaccines in fighting COVID-19 has been promising, leading to interest in their usage for other disorders. In cancer therapy, mRNA may create tumor-associated antigens to help the immune system kill cancer cells. MicroRNAs (mRNA) may replace missing proteins in hereditary disorders. By expressing CRISPR-Cas9 on mRNA, genomic modifications may be precise (Ahmed, 2022; Lorentzen, Haanen, Met, & Svane, 2022).

Despite its potential, mRNA treatment has hurdles. mRNA is unstable and degrades quickly, requiring safe delivery. Manage the immunogenicity of mRNA, which activates the immune system, to reduce risks. Targeting mRNA to particular cells and tissues is difficult, especially in non-vaccine applications. Nevertheless, mRNA treatments have many benefits (Ahmed, 2022; Han, Noh et al., 2023). This kind of medication may be produced and changed quickly to address growing health hazards. Additionally, messenger RNA (mRNA) does not integrate into the genome, lowering the risk of genetic changes. Additionally, mRNA drives powerful but temporary protein synthesis, which may benefit numerous therapeutic applications. Future studies might improve delivery, mRNA stability, and targeting. MicroRNA (mRNA) therapy may assist oncology, infectious illnesses, and unusual genetic disorders. With technology, mRNA treatments may become a major part of contemporary medicine, providing increased accuracy and flexibility in treating numerous illnesses (Lorentzen et al., 2022; Xie et al., 2022).

2.1 Types of mRNA therapies

mRNA therapies represent a promising and innovative approach to treating various diseases (Fig. 1). These therapies harness messenger RNA (mRNA) to instruct cells to produce specific proteins that can either correct a deficiency or provide a therapeutic benefit. Various mRNA therapies as explained in (Table 1), and their respective therapeutic aims dictate their specific uses.

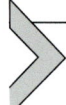

3. Advancements techniques in modifying mRNA for enhanced efficacy

Advancements in mRNA modification techniques aim to enhance the efficacy and therapeutic potential of mRNA-based treatments as shown in Table 2. One key area of improvement is chemical modifications, where nucleotides are altered—such as incorporating pseudouridine or 5-methyl-cytidine—to reduce immune recognition and increase mRNA stability and translation efficiency. Optimizing the 5′ cap structure of mRNA can further improve stability and translation. Delivery systems, such as lipid nanoparticles (LNPs), have also seen significant advancements.

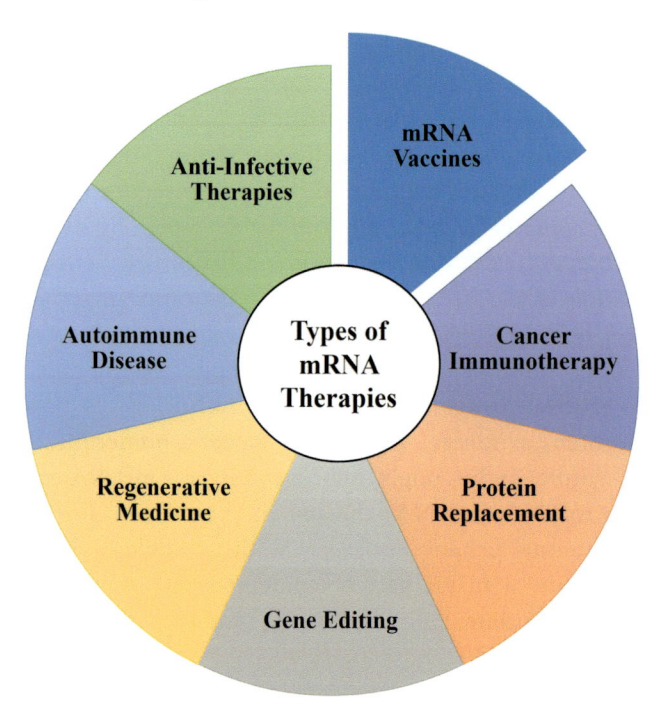

Fig. 1 Types of mRNA therapies.

Table 1 Types of mRNA therapies.

Type	Purpose	Mechanism	Examples/Applications	References
mRNA Vaccines	Stimulate an immune response by encoding specific antigens	mRNA is translated into a protein antigen, prompting the immune system to create antibodies	COVID-19 vaccines (Pfizer-BioNTech, Moderna)	Liu, Yan, Zeng, Fan, and Xiong (2024)
Cancer Immunotherapy	Enhance the immune response against cancer by encoding tumor-associated antigens	mRNA directs cells to produce TAAs, helping the immune system recognize and attack cancer cells	Personalized cancer vaccines targeting tumor mutations	Brandenburg, Heine, and Brossart (2024)
Protein Replacement	Replace missing or defective proteins in genetic disorders	mRNA enables cells to produce functional proteins, restoring normal cellular function	Cystic fibrosis, enzyme deficiencies	Bai, Feng, and Schmid (2024)
Gene Editing	Enable genome editing using mRNA-encoded gene-editing tools	mRNA translates into proteins like Cas9 to edit DNA, correcting genetic mutations	CRISPR-based therapies for genetic disorders	Atsavapranee, Billingsley, and Mitchell (2021)
Regenerative Medicine	Promote tissue repair and regeneration	mRNA encodes growth factors or proteins that stimulate tissue healing	Heart regeneration after heart attacks, muscle injury repair	Kuang, Zhang, Yu, Shang, and Zhao (2023)
Autoimmune Disease	Modulate the immune system to reduce harmful autoimmune responses	mRNA directs the production of regulatory proteins that reduce immune activity	Multiple sclerosis, rheumatoid arthritis	Zhao, Li, Yin, Feng, and Lu (2023)
Anti-Infective Therapies	Fight infections by encoding proteins that attack pathogens	mRNA produces proteins that directly neutralize pathogens or enhance immune defense	Broad applications against viral, bacterial, or parasitic infections	Bertaglia et al. (2023)

Table 2 Advances in mRNA modification techniques.

Modification technique	Purpose	Mechanism	Impact	References
Nucleotide Modifications	Improve mRNA stability and reduce immune activation	Chemical modifications (e.g., pseudouridine, 5-methylcytidine) prevent immune recognition	Enhanced translation efficiency and increased mRNA half-life	Mei and Wang (2023); Wu, Gong et al. (2022)
Cap Structure Optimization	Enhance mRNA translation and stability	Optimizing the 5′ cap structure (e.g., anti-reverse cap analogs) protects mRNA and improves translation	Improved protein production and reduced degradation	Beck et al. (2021); De Mey, Esprit, Thielemans, Breckpot, and Franceschini (2022)
Poly(A) Tail Length Modifications	Control mRNA stability and translation efficiency	Adjusting the length of the poly(A) tail to optimize mRNA stability and translation efficiency	Enhanced protein expression and sustained therapeutic effects	Jalkanen, Coleman, and Wilusz (2014); Kwak, Daly, Fogarty, Grimson, and Kwak (2022)
Untranslated Region (UTR) Engineering	Regulate mRNA translation and stability	Engineering the 5′ and 3′ UTRs to promote efficient translation and protect against degradation	Increased protein output and controlled therapeutic response	Liu et al. (2021); Schuster and Hsieh (2019)
Lipid Nanoparticle (LNP) Enhancements	Improve mRNA delivery and cellular uptake	Optimizing LNP formulations for better mRNA encapsulation and cellular delivery	Higher delivery success rates and more effective mRNA therapies	Han, Lim et al. (2023); Zhang, Yao, Hu, Zhao, and Lee (2022)

Self-amplifying mRNA (saRNA)	Increase protein expression with smaller mRNA doses	mRNA encodes both protein and viral RNA replicase, allowing self-replication inside cells	Greater protein expression with lower doses, reducing cost and side effects	Dailey, Crosby, and Hartman (2023); Papukashvili et al. (2022)
Circular mRNA	Enhance stability and translation	Circular mRNA resists degradation due to the lack of free ends, allowing for sustained translation	Prolonged protein production and increased stability	Li, Peng et al. (2022); Ma, Wang, Zhang, Wang, and Long (2024)
Immune Evasion Strategies	Reduce unwanted immune responses to mRNA	Modifying RNA or delivery methods to avoid triggering innate immune receptors	Lower risk of immune-related side effects, improved safety	Kim and Cho (2022); Vinay et al. (2015)
Targeted Delivery Systems	Direct mRNA to specific tissues or cells	Using tissue-specific ligands on nanoparticles to precisely deliver mRNA to targeted cells/organs	Higher therapeutic efficacy with fewer side effects	Riley, June, Langer, and Mitchell (2019); Yang et al. (2022)

4. Incorporation of immunomodulatory elements

Incorporating immunomodulatory components into mRNA treatments is a complex strategy to improve their effectiveness, especially in cancer treatment. Maximizing the transport and stability of messenger RNA is a primary goal. Chemically modified nucleotides like pseudouridine make mRNA less immune system-recognizable and less degradable. Lipid nanoparticles (LNPs) preserve mRNA during transport and help target cells absorb it (Fig. 2) (Matsushita & Kawaguchi, 2018; Roy, Singh, & Misra, 2022; Wu, Yang, Cheng, Bi, & Chen, 2022).

Another important advance is mRNA vaccines targeting tumor-specific antigens. These vaccines encode tumor-specific proteins. These proteins trigger an immunological response, helping the immune system identify and kill cancer cells while protecting healthy tissue. Personalized mRNA vaccines for neoantigen targeting are improving this method. Neoantigens are unique tumor mutations that can be detected via next-generation sequencing. Create personalized mRNA vaccines that encode these neoantigens for a more targeted and effective immune response against malignancy (Li, Shi et al., 2022).

Combinations of mRNA vaccines and immune checkpoint inhibitors are also garnering interest. Checkpoint inhibitors disrupt proteins like PD-1 and CTLA-4 that hinder T lymphocytes from attacking cancer cells. Using mRNA vaccines to stimulate the immune system with checkpoint inhibitors

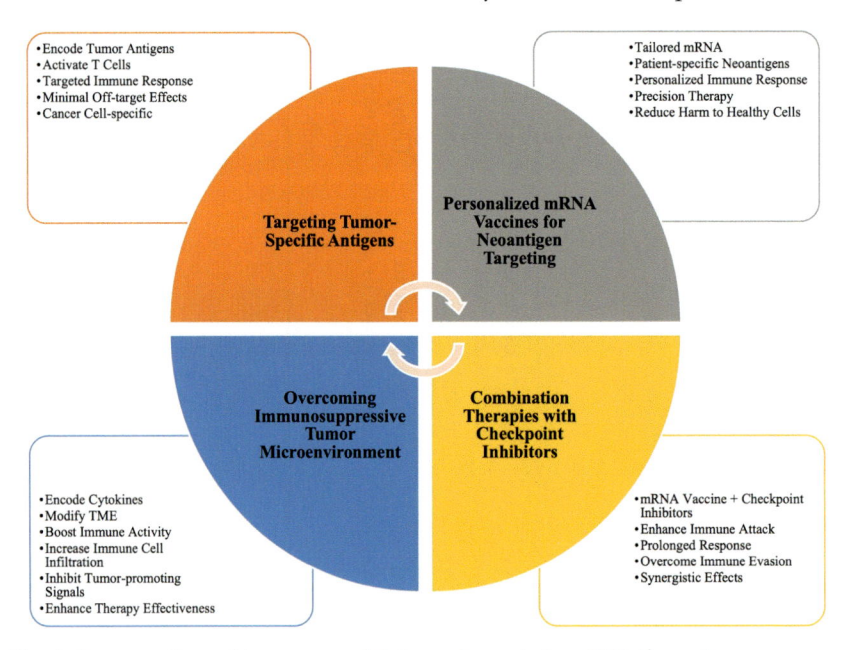

Fig. 2 Incorporation of immunomodulatory elements in mRNA therapies.

to eliminate inhibitory signals creates a synergistic effect that boosts and prolongs anti-tumor responses (Li, Shi et al., 2022; Qiu et al., 2024).

Finally, addressing the immunosuppressive tumor microenvironment with mRNA treatments is difficult. Tumors generally inhibit the immune system, making it hard for the body to fight back. To combat this, researchers are designing mRNA that encodes cytokines or other immunostimulatory molecules to improve the tumor milieu for immune activation. Targeted delivery methods deliver mRNA treatments to the tumor site, where they stimulate the immune response locally (Locy et al., 2018; Zhang & Zhang, 2020).

5. Innovative delivery strategies for mRNA therapies

Innovative delivery strategies are crucial for the success of mRNA therapies, as they address the challenge of effectively transporting mRNA into target cells while minimizing degradation and enhancing specificity. Here are some of the most promising strategies as shown in Table 3.

6. Advancements in mRNA vaccine development

Growth in mRNA vaccine development has broadened its use beyond infectious illnesses to cancer immunotherapy and autoimmune disorders (Zhao et al., 2023). Optimizing mRNA design using codon optimization and changed nucleotides improves stability and protein synthesis, boosting immune responses and reducing adverse effects. Protection of mRNA and cell absorption by advanced delivery technologies like lipid nanoparticles (LNPs) boost vaccination effectiveness and applicability. Self-amplifying mRNA (saRNA) is another important discovery. This method replicates mRNA in cells, decreasing dosage and boosting scalability (Dailey et al., 2023; Papukashvili et al., 2022). Multivalent and combination vaccines, which encode many antigens, provide greater protection with fewer doses, making them beneficial for influenza and combinations in cancer therapy. Customized mRNA vaccines for tumor-specific neoantigens are a breakthrough in precision medicine, notably in cancer treatment (Lorentzen et al., 2022; Samec et al., 2022). Focusing on adjuvants and tailored mRNA boosts immunogenicity, decreasing booster dosages. mRNA vaccines are more stable at warmer temperatures because of cold chain improvements, making worldwide distribution easier, especially in places lacking ultra-cold storage. Finally, mRNA vaccine applications in cancer, autoimmune illnesses, and allergies show its adaptability and transformational promise in contemporary medicine (Table 4) (Duan et al., 2022; Liu et al., 2024; Mei & Wang, 2023).

Table 3 Innovative delivery strategies for mRNA therapies.

Delivery strategy	Purpose	Key features	Advantages	Challenges	Applications	References
Lipid Nanoparticles (LNPs)	Protect mRNA and enhance cellular uptake	Lipid bilayer encapsulation, advanced particle engineering	High efficiency, widely used, improved mRNA stability	Immunogenicity concerns, limited targeting to specific tissues	COVID−19 vaccines, cancer immunotherapy, gene editing	Han, Noh et al. (2023); Hao et al. (2023)
Polymeric Nanoparticles	Versatile and customizable mRNA delivery	Biodegradable polymers (e.g., PLGA), controlled release	Tunable release profiles, biocompatibility, adaptability for various therapies	Manufacturing complexity, the potential toxicity of degradation products	Cancer treatment, gene therapy, vaccines	Xiao et al. (2022); Yu et al. (2023)
Exosome-Mediated Delivery	Use natural vesicles for targeted delivery	Biocompatible exosomes, endogenous vesicle engineering	Ability to cross biological barriers (e.g., blood-brain barrier), low immunogenicity	Difficult to produce at scale, heterogeneity in exosome populations	Neurological disorders, cancer immunotherapy	Roy, Girija AS, Sankar Ganesh, Saravanan, and Sunny (2023); Zhang, Liu et al. (2022)
Peptide-Based Delivery Systems	Enhance cellular uptake and tissue targeting	Short amino acid chains, cell-penetrating peptides	Efficient cellular entry, potential for targeted delivery	Stability and degradation in the bloodstream, immune responses	Cardiovascular diseases, cancer treatment	Guo et al. (2024); Samec, Boulos, Gilmore, Hazelton, and Alexander-Bryant (2022)

Ligand-Conjugated Nanoparticles	Achieve precise delivery to specific cells	Surface ligands (e.g., antibodies, small molecules) for receptor targeting	Specific targeting of diseased tissues reduces off-target effects	Complex design, potential immune responses to ligands	Personalized cancer therapy, targeted gene therapy	Karra and Benita (2012); Yan, Na, Liu, and Wu (2024)
RNA Aptamer-Based Delivery	Improve precision of mRNA delivery	RNA aptamers that bind to specific target molecules	Highly selective targeting minimizes impact on healthy cells	Stability and manufacturing challenges, limited clinical experience	Cancer treatment, precision medicine	Mahmoudian et al. (2024)
Intranasal and Oral Delivery Routes	Provide non-invasive delivery options	Formulations for mucosal surfaces, protection against degradation	Patient-friendly, non-invasive, suitable for large-scale vaccination	Limited bioavailability, challenges with absorption and degradation	Vaccines, respiratory and gastrointestinal disorders	Bruinsmann et al. (2019)
Hydrogel-Based Delivery Systems	Sustain mRNA release at the target site	Water-based gels, environmental triggers (e.g., pH, temperature)	Localized and controlled release, customizable degradation rates	Limited applications for systemic delivery, stability concerns	Tissue engineering, wound healing, cancer therapy	Cui et al. (2021)
Electroporation	Enhance cellular uptake using electric pulses	Temporary increase in cell membrane permeability, equipment-dependent	Efficient mRNA entry into difficult-to-transfect cells (e.g., immune cells)	Requires specialized equipment, potential cell damage due to electric pulses	Gene therapy, vaccine development	Justesen, Orhan, Raskov, Nolsoe, and Gögenur (2022)

Table 4 Advancements in mRNA vaccine development.

Advancement	Description	Impact	Applications	References
Optimized mRNA Design	Sequence optimization, codon optimization, use of modified nucleotides	Higher protein production, improved immune responses, reduced side effects	COVID−19 vaccines, cancer immunotherapy, autoimmune diseases	Mei and Wang (2023)
Advanced Delivery Systems	Improved LNPs and other delivery vehicles	Enhanced mRNA stability, better cellular uptake, reduced toxicity	Broad use in vaccines, gene therapy	Liu et al. (2024)
Self-amplifying mRNA (saRNA)	mRNA replication machinery to amplify antigen production	Lower doses required, reduced production costs, enhanced immune response	Vaccines for low-resource settings, cancer, and infectious diseases	Dailey et al. (2023); Papukashvili et al. (2022)
Multivalent and Combination Vaccines	Vaccines encoding multiple antigens	Broader protection, increased efficiency, fewer injections	Influenza, respiratory diseases, combination cancer-immunotherapy vaccines	Brandenburg et al. (2024); Kuang et al. (2023)
Personalized mRNA Vaccines	Custom vaccines targeting patient-specific tumor neoantigens	Tailored immune responses, more effective cancer treatment	Cancer immunotherapy, precision medicine	Riley et al. (2019)

Enhancing Immunogenicity	Incorporation of adjuvants, engineering mRNA for stronger immune activation	Stronger and longer-lasting immune responses, fewer boosters required	Vaccines for older adults, immunocompromised individuals	Matsushita and Kawaguchi (2018); Riley et al. (2019)
Cold Chain Improvements	Development of mRNA vaccines stable at higher temperatures	Expanded distribution, increased accessibility	Global vaccine distribution, especially in low-resource regions	Ma et al. (2024)
Broadened Applications Beyond Infectious Diseases	mRNA vaccines for cancer, autoimmune diseases, allergies	New treatment approaches, precision medicine	Cancer treatment, autoimmune disease modulation, allergen-specific immunotherapy	Bertaglia et al. (2023); Zhang and Zhang (2020)

6.1 COVID-19 mRNA vaccines as a case study

Technology and public health advanced with the development and use of mRNA vaccines during the COVID-19 pandemic. Pfizer-BioNTech and Moderna's mRNA vaccines were the first to be authorized for general use and illustrated how this technology may impact global health. This case study highlights the COVID-19 mRNA vaccine development's speed. Unlike conventional vaccinations, mRNA vaccines were designed, tested, and distributed in less than a year. Modern mRNA technology, including optimized sequences, improved delivery mechanisms, and the ability to target new viral strains, permitted this quick turnaround. Human cells get SARS-CoV-2 spike protein mRNA from COVID-19 mRNA vaccinations (Krause, 2023; Shroff et al., 2021). Cells transcribe mRNA into spike protein to make antibodies and activate T cells. The body can detect and fight illness if exposed. mRNA vaccines reduce pathogen handling risks, unlike live or inactivated viral vaccines. Clinical trials show that mRNA COVID-19 vaccines reduce symptomatic illness by 94–95 %. These vaccines also reduce breakthrough illness severity. Moderate and temporary side effects include injection site pain and flu-like symptoms. Immunization advantages outweigh risks like myocarditis. Scalability was essential for mRNA vaccine production to meet global demand. mRNA vaccines may be mass-produced owing to their synthetic nature and biomanufacturing advances. Early challenges included ultra-cold storage at −70 °C for the Pfizer-BioNTech vaccine (Barbier, Jiang, Zhang, Wooster, & Anderson, 2022; Miao, Zhang, & Huang, 2021). Recently developed vaccinations are more stable at higher temperatures, simplifying delivery. The COVID-19 mRNA vaccine has saved millions of lives. Immunizations have decreased healthcare expenses, public health limitations, and economic development. Successful mRNA COVID-19 vaccines have prompted research into mRNA technology for additional diseases, including new SARS-CoV-2 variants, influenza, and cancer. The success of mRNA COVID-19 vaccines has several lessons for future research. First, mRNA's diversity and speed make it suitable for infectious disease development. Public-private alliances and regulatory agility speed vaccine development amid health emergencies. Finally, better vaccine storage and distribution may help epidemic logistics (Fig. 3) (Krause, 2023; Miao et al., 2021; Ruiz, Lopez-Olivo, Geng, & Suarez-Almazor, 2023). Details of COVID-19 vaccine platform has been mentioned in Table 5.

Responses to the COVID-19 Vaccine in the Immune System

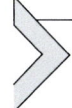

Fig. 3 Response to the COVID-19 vaccines in the immune system.

7. Clinical trials and progress in mRNA-based cancer immunotherapies

mRNA-based cancer immunotherapies are potential ways to use the immune system to kill cancer cells. These medicines use mRNA to encode tumor antigens to trigger an immune response that kills cancer cells. Multiple clinical studies and early triumphs have advanced this discipline (Table 6).

Table 5 COVID-19 vaccine platforms.

Vaccine type	Mechanism of action	Advantages	Challenges	Efficacy	Dosing	Storage	Approved/ prominent examples	Applications	References
mRNA Vaccines	Synthetic mRNA encodes viral protein; cells produce antigen	Rapid development High efficacy Adaptable to variants No risk of live virus infection	Cold-chain storage Rare side effects (e.g., myocarditis) Short-term reactogenicity	~94–95 % against symptomatic COVID−19	2 doses (booster recommended)	Ultra-cold storage (−70 °C) initially, now more stable at 2–8 °C	Pfizer-BioNTech (Comirnaty), Moderna (Spikevax)	Global vaccination campaigns, future pandemics, cancer vaccines	Krause (2023); Shroff et al. (2021)
Adenoviral Vector Vaccines	Adenovirus delivers DNA encoding viral protein	Robust immune response T-cell activation Stable at regular refrigerator temps Single-dose option	Lower efficacy compared to mRNA Rare blood clotting disorders Pre-existing immunity to vectors can reduce efficacy	~70–85 % against symptomatic COVID−19	Single-dose or 2 doses (booster required)	Regular refrigerator temperature (2–8 °C)	AstraZeneca (Vaxzevria), Johnson & Johnson (Janssen), Sputnik V	Vaccination in areas with limited cold-chain infrastructure	Chavda et al. (2023); Okuyama (2023)
Protein-Based Vaccines	Pre-formed viral proteins delivered directly, often with adjuvants	Established technology Safer profile Stable storage Lower side effect risk Less reactogenic	Slower to develop May need adjuvants or multiple doses Lower immunogenicity	~89–90 % against symptomatic COVID−19	2 doses (booster required)	Regular refrigerator temperature (2–8 °C)	Novavax (Nuvaxovid), Sanofi-GSK	Suitable for vaccine-hesitant populations, Global vaccination	Jalkanen et al. (2014); Papukashvili et al. (2022)

Vaccine type	Mechanism	Advantages	Disadvantages	Efficacy	Dosage	Storage	Manufacturers	Applications	References
Attenuated Virus Vaccines	Weakened live virus stimulates a broad immune response	Mimics natural infection Provides broad and long-lasting immunity Often single-dose Elicits strong mucosal immunity	Complex manufacturing Risk of reversion to virulence Not for immunocompromised individuals Safety concerns in pregnant women	Varies depending on the strain, generally effective	Single-dose, possible boosters	Cold storage (2–8 °C)	Codagenix, Bharat Biotech (Covaxin)	High-risk populations, broader immunity coverage	Li et al. (2023); Wei and Hui (2022)
Inactivated Virus Vaccines	Killed virus used to stimulate immune response	A long history of use Stable Well-understood mechanism Lower risk of adverse events	Weaker immune response May require boosters Slower to produce in large quantities	~50–78 % against symptomatic COVID−19	2 doses (booster required)	Regular refrigerator temperature (2–8 °C)	Sinopharm, Sinovac (CoronaVac)	Broad use in countries with traditional vaccine infrastructure	Hayashi and Konishi (2023); Wang, Pei, Xu, Liu, and Yu (2023)
DNA Vaccines	Plasmid DNA encodes a viral protein, delivered to cells	Stable at room temperature Cost-effective Easy to manufacture No live virus handling	Lower immunogenicity Requires electroporation for delivery Limited real-world data	Early data shows moderate efficacy	Multiple doses may be needed	Regular refrigerator temperature (2–8 °C)	Zydus Cadila (ZyCoV-D)	Emerging technology for pandemic preparedness, potential booster applications	Goyal et al. (2023); Katopodi et al. (2024)

Table 6 Clinical trials and progress in mRNA-based cancer immunotherapies.

Therapy type	Approach	Current clinical trials	Outcomes/impact	Challenges	References
Personalized mRNA Vaccines	Vaccines tailored to patient-specific tumor neoantigens, identified through tumor sequencing.	BioNTech & Moderna trials for melanoma, NSCLC, ovarian cancer, breast cancer.	Strong immune responses and early tumor regression were observed and well-tolerated in various cancers.	High-cost, complex logistics for patient-specific manufacturing.	Donhauser et al. (2023)
Off-the-Shelf mRNA Vaccines	Vaccines targeting common cancer-associated antigens applicable to a broader population.	KRAS-mutated pancreatic, colorectal, and lung cancer trials; HPV+ cervical cancer studies.	Broad applicability, faster production; and potential to target frequent mutations in multiple cancer types.	Limited effectiveness in highly heterogeneous tumors.	Ni (2023)
Combination Therapies	Combining mRNA vaccines with immune checkpoint inhibitors (e.g., PD−1/PD-L1 blockers).	Trials for melanoma, NSCLC, bladder cancer, and renal cell carcinoma (RCC).	Increased overall survival, stronger immune response, and reduction in tumor size were observed.	Managing enhanced toxicity from combined therapies, treatment resistance.	Brandenburg et al. (2024);Kuang et al. (2023)
mRNA-Based Adoptive Cell Therapies	Engineering T cells with mRNA to express receptors targeting tumor-specific antigens (e.g., CAR-T).	Blood cancers (leukemia, lymphoma) and solid tumors (glioblastoma, ovarian cancer, mesothelioma).	High precision targeting, improved durability of response, and potential to treat resistant cancers.	Difficulty in targeting solid tumors, off-target effects, and managing cytokine release syndrome (CRS).	Krause (2023)
Self-amplifying mRNA (saRNA)	Prolonged antigen expression via saRNA technology for a stronger and longer immune response.	Early trials in melanoma, glioblastoma, and liver cancer; preclinical studies in breast and colorectal cancers.	Higher potency with smaller doses, sustained immune activation, enhanced cost-effectiveness.	Risk of prolonged inflammation, scalability of production, and delivery challenges in certain cancers.	Dailey et al. (2023); Papukashvili et al. (2022)

Approach	Description	Applications/Trials	Benefits	Challenges	References
Tumor Microenvironment Modulation	mRNA therapies to modulate the tumor microenvironment, enhancing immune responses against tumors.	Pancreatic, ovarian, and gastric cancer trials; preclinical studies on immune-modulatory cytokines like IL-12, GM-CSF.	Overcomes immune suppression in the TME, synergizes with other therapies, and improves response rates.	The complexity of reprogramming the TME, the risk of triggering excessive immune responses, and limited biomarkers.	Kim and Cho (2022); Locy et al. (2018)
Neoantigen Targeting with mRNA	mRNA vaccines targeting patient-specific neoantigens for a highly personalized immune response.	Neoantigen trials in breast, colorectal, and lung cancers; Moderna's individualized cancer vaccine project (Vaccine No. V941).	Improved progression-free survival (PFS); is particularly effective for cancers with high mutational burden.	Identification of actionable neoantigens, time, and cost of individual sequencing.	Imani, Tagit, and Pichon (2024)
Oncolytic mRNA Therapy	mRNA encoding proteins that directly kill cancer cells or stimulate immune responses to tumors.	Preclinical and early-phase trials in glioma, melanoma, and prostate cancer using oncolytic virus vectors delivering mRNA.	Direct tumor cell killing, and enhanced immune infiltration into tumors, promising in combination with immune checkpoint blockade.	Risk of off-target effects, delivery to the tumor site, and challenges with systemic administration.	Bertaglia et al. (2023); Wei and Hui (2022)
mRNA-Induced Cytokine Therapies	mRNA vaccines are designed to produce cytokines that stimulate the immune system to attack tumors.	Trials for melanoma, head and neck cancers, and metastatic cancers involving cytokines like IL-2, and GM-CSF.	Potent immune activation, improved survival in some patients, synergistic with checkpoint inhibitors.	Potential for severe inflammatory side effects, dose-limiting toxicities, and need for precise delivery.	Krause (2023); Ni (2023)

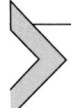

8. Challenges and future directions in mRNA therapies for cancer immunotherapy

8.1 Overcoming barriers to delivery and translation into clinical practice (Table 7)

Table 7 Overcoming barriers to mRNA therapy delivery and emerging strategies.

Challenge	Strategy/ technology	Description	Outcome	References
Delivery Efficiency	Next-Generation Nanoparticles	Smaller, flexible nanoparticles with targeted delivery to tumor cells.	Improved precision in targeting tumors, and reduced off-target effects.	Riley et al. (2019); Yang et al. (2022)
Tumor Heterogeneity	Multivalent & Personalized mRNA Vaccines	Vaccines targeting multiple antigens or personalized to specific tumor neoantigens.	Broader coverage of diverse tumor cell populations, and tailored therapy for individual patients.	Katopodi et al. (2024); Zhang and Zhang (2020)
Modulating Tumor Microenvironment (TME)	Combination Therapies & Immune-Modulatory mRNA	Combining vaccines with checkpoint inhibitors or encoding immune-enhancing cytokines in mRNA.	Reprogrammed TME, improved immune response within the tumor.	Kim and Cho (2022); Locy et al. (2018)
Immunogenicity & Side Effects	Modified Nucleosides in mRNA	Incorporating modified nucleosides (e.g., pseudouridine) to prevent excessive immune activation.	Reduced inflammation, and balanced immune activation for safer therapy.	Matsushita and Kawaguchi (2018); Roy et al. (2022)
Scaling Up Manufacturing & Global Access	Automation, Synthetic Biology & Temperature-Stable Formulations	Streamlined production processes and formulations that don't require cold storage.	Cost-effective manufacturing, and improved access in low-resource settings.	Bertaglia et al. (2023)

Self-amplifying mRNA (saRNA)	Self-Amplifying mRNA	mRNA that replicates within cells, reducing the required dose.	Enhanced immune response with smaller doses, cost reduction.	Dailey et al. (2023); Papukashvili et al. (2022)
Neoantigen Targeting	Personalized Neoantigen Vaccines	mRNA vaccines targeting tumor-specific neoantigens identified through sequencing.	Stronger, more precise immune responses, especially in cancers like melanoma.	Imani et al. (2024)
Oncolytic mRNA Therapies	Oncolytic mRNA	mRNA encoding proteins that kill cancer cells or stimulate immune responses.	Promising early results in treating solid tumors resistant to other immunothera-pies.	Wei and Hui (2022)
Combination Therapies	Combining mRNA Vaccines with Immune Checkpoint Inhibitors, CAR-T, Radiation	Using mRNA vaccines alongside other cancer therapies to boost efficacy.	Enhanced treatment response, particularly in resistant cancers such as NSCLC and melanoma.	Brandenburg et al. (2024); Kuang et al. (2023)
Advances in Delivery Systems	Polymer-Based Nanoparticles, Cell-Penetrating Peptides, Hybrid Systems	Novel materials and systems for improved mRNA stability and tumor penetration.	Increased delivery efficiency and effectiveness, particularly in hard-to-reach tumors.	Riley et al. (2019); Roy et al. (2022)
Immune Tuning & Safety Enhancements	Optimized Adjuvants & Engineered mRNA Sequences	Fine-tuning immune response to avoid excessive inflammation while maintaining efficacy.	Safer therapies with balanced immune activation, reduce the risk of side effects such as cytokine release syndrome.	Vinay et al. (2015); Wu, Gong et al. (2022)

9. Conclusion (summary and outlook: future therapy)

Over the past few decades, mRNA nanomedicines have demonstrated amazing beneficial properties, making them potential candidates for the creation of a variety of novel treatments. These characteristics include the lack of genotoxicity hazards, the capacity to target non-drug targets, flexibility in manipulation, cost-effectiveness, and quick large-scale production.

The incredible effectiveness of immunotherapy has shown that the immune system is still one of our most potent cancer-fighting capabilities. To improve anti-cancer immune responses, researchers and clinicians must work together to expand our understanding of tumor immunology, innovative therapy modalities, and delivery strategies.

mRNA regarded as potential remedial as well as medicinal component in order to cure and avoid a variety of disorders, like cancer, because of its regulated and temporary expression of protein characteristics. In comparison to DNA-based treatments, mRNA posses greater safety nature since it does'nt need to be localized towards nucleus, reducing the danger for genetic alteration. Thus, the unstable gentic phenomenon, immunogenicity, along with limited transport effectiveness of negatively charged RNA limit its use in cancer treatment. Moreover, immune checkpoint therapy, radiation, chemotherapy, and therapy combinations with mRNA-based cancer vaccines may enhance the efficacy and responsiveness of treatments.

The mRNA possesses enormous biological promise as a therapeutic component for a variety of utilization, such as vaccinations of cancer. Current research defines significant advances for mRNA treatments in a variety of therapeutic techniques, including cancer immunotherapy, vaccinations, replacement of protein replacement, and genetic modification. Considering a number of pharmacological and biological barriers requiring to be addressed prior clinical applications, latest advancements like mRNA vaccines against COVID-19 and other treatments for clinical trials demonstrate mRNA's potential as a game-changing treatment for a variety of disorders. We anticipate that continued attempts to innovate and optimize mRNA technology will yield innovative and beneficial results in life science and medical research.

References

Ahmed, T. (2022). Immunotherapy for neuroblastoma using mRNA vaccines. *Advances in Cancer Biology − Metastasis, 4*, 100033. https://doi.org/10.1016/j.adcanc.2022.100033.

Atsavapranee, E. S., Billingsley, M. M., & Mitchell, M. J. (2021). Delivery technologies for T cell gene editing: Applications in cancer immunotherapy. *EBioMedicine, 67*, 103354. https://doi.org/10.1016/j.ebiom.2021.103354.

Bai, H., Feng, L., & Schmid, F. (2024). Macrophage-based cancer immunotherapy: Challenges and opportunities. *Experimental Cell Research, 442*, 114198. https://doi.org/10.1016/j.yexcr.2024.114198.

Barbier, A. J., Jiang, A. Y., Zhang, P., Wooster, R., & Anderson, D. G. (2022). The clinical progress of mRNA vaccines and immunotherapies. *Nature Biotechnology, 40*, 840–854. https://doi.org/10.1038/s41587-022-01294-2.

Beck, J. D., Reidenbach, D., Salomon, N., Sahin, U., Türeci, Ö., Vormehr, M., & Kranz, L. M. (2021). mRNA therapeutics in cancer immunotherapy. *Molecular Cancer, 20*, 69. https://doi.org/10.1186/s12943-021-01348-0.

Bertaglia, V., Morelli, A. M., Solinas, C., Aiello, M. M., Manunta, S., Denaro, N., ... Novello, S. (2023). Infections in lung cancer patients undergoing immunotherapy and targeted therapy: An overview on the current scenario. *Critical Reviews in Oncology/Hematology, 184*, 103954. https://doi.org/10.1016/j.critrevonc.2023.103954.

Brandenburg, A., Heine, A., & Brossart, P. (2024). Next-generation cancer vaccines and emerging immunotherapy combinations. *Trends Cancer, 10*, 749–769. https://doi.org/10.1016/j.trecan.2024.06.003.

Bruinsmann, F. A., Richter Vaz, G., de Cristo Soares Alves, A., Aguirre, T., Raffin Pohlmann, A., Stanisçuaski Guterres, S., & Sonvico, F. (2019). Nasal drug delivery of anticancer drugs for the treatment of glioblastoma: Preclinical and clinical trials. *Molecules (Basel, Switzerland), 24*, 4312. https://doi.org/10.3390/molecules24234312.

Chavda, V., Bezbaruah, R., Valu, D., Patel, B., Kumar, A., Prasad, S., ... Jesawadawala, M. (2023). Adenoviral vector-based vaccine platform for COVID-19: Current status. *Vaccines (Basel), 11*, 432. https://doi.org/10.3390/vaccines11020432.

Cui, R., Wu, Q., Wang, J., Zheng, X., Ou, R., Xu, Y., ... Li, D. (2021). Hydrogel-by-design: Smart delivery system for cancer immunotherapy. *Frontiers in Bioengineering and Biotechnology, 9*. https://doi.org/10.3389/fbioe.2021.723490.

Dailey, G. P., Crosby, E. J., & Hartman, Z. C. (2023). Cancer vaccine strategies using self-replicating RNA viral platforms. *Cancer Gene Therapy, 30*, 794–802. https://doi.org/10.1038/s41417-022-00499-6.

De Mey, W., Esprit, A., Thielemans, K., Breckpot, K., & Franceschini, L. (2022). RNA in cancer immunotherapy: Unlocking the potential of the immune system. *Clinical Cancer Research: An Official Journal of the American Association for Cancer Research, 28*, 3929–3939. https://doi.org/10.1158/1078-0432.CCR-21-3304.

Donhauser, L. V., Veloso de Oliveira, J., Schick, C., Manlik, W., Styblova, S., Lutzenberger, S., ... Zehn, D. (2023). Responses of patients with cancer to mRNA vaccines depend on the time interval between vaccination and last treatment. *The Journal for ImmunoTherapy of Cancer, 11*, e007387. https://doi.org/10.1136/jitc-2023-007387.

Duan, L.-J., Wang, Q., Zhang, C., Yang, D.-X., & Zhang, X.-Y. (2022). Potentialities and challenges of mRNA vaccine in cancer immunotherapy. *Frontiers in Immunology, 13*. https://doi.org/10.3389/fimmu.2022.923647.

Goyal, F., Chattopadhyay, A., Navik, U., Jain, A., Reddy, P. H., Bhatti, G. K., & Bhatti, J. S. (2023). Advancing cancer immunotherapy: The potential of mRNA vaccines as a promising therapeutic approach. *Advances in Therapy (Weinh)*. https://doi.org/10.1002/adtp.202300255.

Guo, S., Wang, J., Wang, Q., Wang, J., Qin, S., & Li, W. (2024). Advances in peptide-based drug delivery systems. *Heliyon, 10*, e26009. https://doi.org/10.1016/j.heliyon.2024.e26009.

Han, J., Lim, J., Wang, C.-P. J., Han, J.-H., Shin, H. E., Kim, S.-N., ... Park, W. (2023). Lipid nanoparticle-based mRNA delivery systems for cancer immunotherapy. *Nano Convergence, 10*, 36. https://doi.org/10.1186/s40580-023-00385-3.

Han, G., Noh, D., Lee, H., Lee, S., Kim, S., Yoon, H. Y., & Lee, S. H. (2023). Advances in mRNA therapeutics for cancer immunotherapy: From modification to delivery. *Advanced Drug Delivery Reviews, 199*, 114973. https://doi.org/10.1016/j.addr.2023.114973.

Hao, Y., Ji, Z., Zhou, H., Wu, D., Gu, Z., Wang, D., & ten Dijke, P. (2023). Lipid-based nanoparticles as drug delivery systems for cancer immunotherapy. *MedComm (Beijing), 4*. https://doi.org/10.1002/mco2.339.

Hayashi, T., & Konishi, I. (2023). The effect of mRNA-based COVID-19 vaccination on anti-programmed cell death protein 1 blockade for nasopharyngeal cancer may differ from a virus-inactivated vaccine. *World Journal of Clinical Oncology, 14*, 316–320. https://doi.org/10.14740/wjon1620.

Imani, S., Tagit, O., & Pichon, C. (2024). Neoantigen vaccine nanoformulations based on Chemically synthesized minimal mRNA (CmRNA): Small molecules, big impact. *NPJ Vaccines, 9*, 14. https://doi.org/10.1038/s41541-024-00807-1.

Jalkanen, A. L., Coleman, S. J., & Wilusz, J. (2014). Determinants and implications of mRNA poly(A) tail size – Does this protein make my tail look big? *Seminars in Cell & Developmental Biology, 34*, 24–32. https://doi.org/10.1016/j.semcdb.2014.05.018.

Justesen, T. F., Orhan, A., Raskov, H., Nolsoe, C., & Gögenur, I. (2022). Electroporation and immunotherapy—Unleashing the abscopal effect. *Cancers (Basel), 14*, 2876. https://doi.org/10.3390/cancers14122876.

Karra, N., & Benita, S. (2012). The ligand nanoparticle conjugation approach for targeted cancer therapy. *Current Drug Metabolism, 13*, 22–41. https://doi.org/10.2174/138920012798356899.

Katopodi, T., Petanidis, S., Grigoriadou, E., Anestakis, D., Charalampidis, C., Chatziprodromidou, I., ... Kosmidis, C. (2024). Immune specific and tumor-dependent mRNA vaccines for cancer immunotherapy: Reprogramming clinical translation into tumor editing therapy. *Pharmaceutics, 16*, 455. https://doi.org/10.3390/pharmaceutics16040455.

Kim, S. K., & Cho, S. W. (2022). The evasion mechanisms of cancer immunity and drug intervention in the tumor microenvironment. *Frontiers in Pharmacology, 13*, 868695. https://doi.org/10.3389/fphar.2022.868695.

Kong, B., Kim, Y., Kim, E. H., Suk, J. S., & Yang, Y. (2023). mRNA: A promising platform for cancer immunotherapy. *Advanced Drug Delivery Reviews, 199*, 114993. https://doi.org/10.1016/j.addr.2023.114993.

Krause, W. (2023). mRNA—From COVID-19 treatment to cancer immunotherapy. *Biomedicines, 11*, 308. https://doi.org/10.3390/biomedicines11020308.

Kuang, G., Zhang, Q., Yu, Y., Shang, L., & Zhao, Y. (2023). Cryo-shocked cancer cell microgels for tumor postoperative combination immunotherapy and tissue regeneration. *Bioactive Materials, 28*, 326–336. https://doi.org/10.1016/j.bioactmat.2023.05.021.

Kwak, Y., Daly, C. W. P., Fogarty, E. A., Grimson, A., & Kwak, H. (2022). Dynamic and widespread control of poly(A) tail length during macrophage activation. *RNA (New York, N. Y.), 28*, 947–971. https://doi.org/10.1261/rna.078918.121.

Li, H., Peng, K., Yang, K., Ma, W., Qi, S., Yu, X., ... Yu, G. (2022). Circular RNA cancer vaccines drive immunity in hard-to-treat malignancies. *Theranostics, 12*, 6422–6436. https://doi.org/10.7150/thno.77350.

Li, Q., Shi, Z., Zhang, F., Zeng, W., Zhu, D., & Mei, L. (2022). Symphony of nano-materials and immunotherapy based on the cancer–immunity cycle. *Acta Pharmaceutica Sinica B, 12*, 107–134. https://doi.org/10.1016/j.apsb.2021.05.031.

Li, Y., Wang, M., Peng, X., Yang, Y., Chen, Q., Liu, J., ... Li, X. (2023). mRNA vaccine in cancer therapy: Current advance and future outlook. *Clinical and Translational Medicine, 13*. https://doi.org/10.1002/ctm2.1384.

Liu, X., Huang, X., Ma, J., Li, L., Hu, H., Feng, J., ... Liu, L. (2021). 3′untranslated regions (3′UTR) of Gelsolin mRNA displays anticancer effects in non-small cell lung cancer (NSCLC) cells. *American Journal of Cancer Research, 11*, 3857–3876.

Liu, Y., Yan, Q., Zeng, Z., Fan, C., & Xiong, W. (2024). Advances and prospects of mRNA vaccines in cancer immunotherapy. *Biochimica et Biophysica Acta (BBA) – Reviews on Cancer, 1879*, 189068. https://doi.org/10.1016/j.bbcan.2023.189068.

Locy, H., de Mey, S., de Mey, W., De Ridder, M., Thielemans, K., & Maenhout, S. K. (2018). Immunomodulation of the tumor microenvironment: Turn foe into friend. *Frontiers in Immunology, 9*. https://doi.org/10.3389/fimmu.2018.02909.

Lorentzen, C. L., Haanen, J. B., Met, Ö., & Svane, I. M. (2022). Clinical advances and ongoing trials of mRNA vaccines for cancer treatment. *The Lancet Oncology, 23*, e450–e458. https://doi.org/10.1016/S1470-2045(22)00372-2.

Ma, Y., Wang, T., Zhang, X., Wang, P., & Long, F. (2024). The role of circular RNAs in regulating resistance to cancer immunotherapy: Mechanisms and implications. *Cell Death & Disease, 15*, 312. https://doi.org/10.1038/s41419-024-06698-3.

Mahmoudian, F., Ahmari, A., Shabani, S., Sadeghi, B., Fahimirad, S., & Fattahi, F. (2024). Aptamers as an approach to targeted cancer therapy. *Cancer Cell International, 24*, 108. https://doi.org/10.1186/s12935-024-03295-4.

Matsushita, M., & Kawaguchi, M. (2018). Immunomodulatory effects of drugs for effective cancer immunotherapy. *Journal of Oncology, 2018*, 8653489. https://doi.org/10.1155/2018/8653489.

Mei, Y., & Wang, X. (2023). RNA modification in mRNA cancer vaccines. *Clinical and Experimental Medicine, 23*, 1917–1931. https://doi.org/10.1007/s10238-023-01020-5.

Miao, L., Zhang, Y., & Huang, L. (2021). mRNA vaccine for cancer immunotherapy. *Molecular Cancer, 20*, 41. https://doi.org/10.1186/s12943-021-01335-5.

Ni, L. (2023). Advances in mRNA-based cancer vaccines. *Vaccines (Basel), 11*, 1599. https://doi.org/10.3390/vaccines11101599.

Okuyama, R. (2023). mRNA and adenoviral vector vaccine platforms utilized in COVID-19 vaccines: Technologies, ecosystem, and future directions. *Vaccines (Basel), 11*, 1737. https://doi.org/10.3390/vaccines11121737.

Pan, S., Fan, R., Han, B., Tong, A., & Guo, G. (2024). The potential of mRNA vaccines in cancer nanomedicine and immunotherapy. *Trends in Immunology, 45*, 20–31. https://doi.org/10.1016/j.it.2023.11.003.

Papukashvili, D., Rcheulishvili, N., Liu, C., Ji, Y., He, Y., & Wang, P. G. (2022). Self-amplifying RNA approach for protein replacement therapy. *International Journal of Molecular Sciences, 23*. https://doi.org/10.3390/ijms232112884.

Qiu, J., Cheng, Z., Jiang, Z., Gan, L., Zhang, Z., & Xie, Z. (2024). Immunomodulatory precision: A narrative review exploring the critical role of immune checkpoint inhibitors in cancer treatment. *International Journal of Molecular Sciences, 25*, 5490. https://doi.org/10.3390/ijms25105490.

Riley, R. S., June, C. H., Langer, R., & Mitchell, M. J. (2019). Delivery technologies for cancer immunotherapy. *Nature Reviews. Drug Discovery, 18*, 175–196. https://doi.org/10.1038/s41573-018-0006-z.

Roy, A., Girija AS, S., Sankar Ganesh, P., Saravanan, M., & Sunny, B. (2023). Exosome mediated cancer therapeutic approach: Present status and future prospectives. *Asian

Pacific Journal of Cancer Prevention, 24, 363–373. https://doi.org/10.31557/APJCP.2023.24.2.363.

Roy, R., Singh, S. K., & Misra, S. (2022). Advancements in cancer immunotherapies. *Vaccines (Basel), 11.* https://doi.org/10.3390/vaccines11010059.

Ruiz, J. I., Lopez-Olivo, M. A., Geng, Y., & Suarez-Almazor, M. E. (2023). COVID-19 vaccination in patients with cancer receiving immune checkpoint inhibitors: A systematic review and meta-analysis. *The Journal for ImmunoTherapy of Cancer, 11,* e006246. https://doi.org/10.1136/jitc-2022-006246.

Samec, T., Boulos, J., Gilmore, S., Hazelton, A., & Alexander-Bryant, A. (2022). Peptide-based delivery of therapeutics in cancer treatment. *Mater Today Bio, 14,* 100248. https://doi.org/10.1016/j.mtbio.2022.100248.

Schuster, S. L., & Hsieh, A. C. (2019). The untranslated regions of mRNAs in cancer. *Trends Cancer, 5,* 245–262. https://doi.org/10.1016/j.trecan.2019.02.011.

Shroff, R. T., Chalasani, P., Wei, R., Pennington, D., Quirk, G., Schoenle, M. V., ... Bhattacharya, D. (2021). Immune responses to COVID-19 mRNA vaccines in patients with solid tumors on active, immunosuppressive cancer therapy. *medRxiv.* https://doi.org/10.1101/2021.05.13.21257129.

Vinay, D. S., Ryan, E. P., Pawelec, G., Talib, W. H., Stagg, J., Elkord, E., ... Kwon, B. S. (2015). Immune evasion in cancer: Mechanistic basis and therapeutic strategies. *Seminars in Cancer Biology, 35,* S185–S198. https://doi.org/10.1016/j.semcancer.2015.03.004.

Wang, B., Pei, J., Xu, S., Liu, J., & Yu, J. (2023). Recent advances in mRNA cancer vaccines: Meeting challenges and embracing opportunities. *Frontiers in Immunology, 14.* https://doi.org/10.3389/fimmu.2023.1246682.

Wei, J., & Hui, A.-M. (2022). The paradigm shift in treatment from Covid-19 to oncology with mRNA vaccines. *Cancer Treatment Reviews, 107,* 102405. https://doi.org/10.1016/j.ctrv.2022.102405.

Wu, H., Gong, Y., Ji, P., Xie, Y., Jiang, Y.-Z., & Liu, G. (2022). Targeting nucleotide metabolism: A promising approach to enhance cancer immunotherapy. *Journal of Hematology & Oncology, 15,* 45. https://doi.org/10.1186/s13045-022-01263-x.

Wu, Y., Yang, Z., Cheng, K., Bi, H., & Chen, J. (2022). Small molecule-based immunomodulators for cancer therapy. *Acta Pharmaceutica Sinica B, 12,* 4287–4308. https://doi.org/10.1016/j.apsb.2022.11.007.

Xiao, X., Teng, F., Shi, C., Chen, J., Wu, S., Wang, B., ... Li, W. (2022). Polymeric nanoparticles—Promising carriers for cancer therapy. *Frontiers in Bioengineering and Biotechnology, 10.* https://doi.org/10.3389/fbioe.2022.1024143.

Xie, X., Song, T., Feng, Y., Zhang, H., Yang, G., Wu, C., ... Yang, H. (2022). Nanotechnology-based multifunctional vaccines for cancer immunotherapy. *Chemical Engineering Journal, 437,* 135505. https://doi.org/10.1016/j.cej.2022.135505.

Yan, S., Na, J., Liu, X., & Wu, P. (2024). Different targeting ligands-mediated drug delivery systems for tumor therapy. *Pharmaceutics, 16,* 248. https://doi.org/10.3390/pharmaceutics16020248.

Yang, M., Olaoba, O. T., Zhang, C., Kimchi, E. T., Staveley-O'Carroll, K. F., & Li, G. (2022). Cancer immunotherapy and delivery system: An update. *Pharmaceutics, 14.* https://doi.org/10.3390/pharmaceutics14081630.

Yu, Z., Shen, X., Yu, H., Tu, H., Chittasupho, C., & Zhao, Y. (2023). Smart polymeric nanoparticles in cancer immunotherapy. *Pharmaceutics, 15.* https://doi.org/10.3390/pharmaceutics15030775.

Zhang, Y., Liu, Q., Zhang, X., Huang, H., Tang, S., Chai, Y., ... Yang, C. (2022). Recent advances in exosome-mediated nucleic acid delivery for cancer therapy. *Journal of Nanobiotechnology, 20,* 279. https://doi.org/10.1186/s12951-022-01472-z.

Zhang, Y., & Zhang, Z. (2020). The history and advances in cancer immunotherapy: Understanding the characteristics of tumor-infiltrating immune cells and their therapeutic implications. *Cellular & Molecular Immunology, 17*, 807–821. https://doi.org/10.1038/s41423-020-0488-6.

Zhang, Z., Yao, S., Hu, Y., Zhao, X., & Lee, R. J. (2022). Application of lipid-based nanoparticles in cancer immunotherapy. *Frontiers in Immunology, 13*. https://doi.org/10.3389/fimmu.2022.967505.

Zhao, J., Li, L., Yin, H., Feng, X., & Lu, Q. (2023). TIGIT: An emerging immune checkpoint target for immunotherapy in autoimmune disease and cancer. *International Immunopharmacology, 120*, 110358. https://doi.org/10.1016/j.intimp.2023.110358.

mRNA-based cancer vaccines: A novel approach to melanoma treatment

Pranav Kumar Prabhakar[a,*], Tarun Kumar Upadhyay[b], and Sanjeev Kumar Sahu[c]

[a]Department of Biotechnology, School of Engineering and Technology, Nagaland University, Meriema, Kohima, Nagaland, India
[b]Parul Institute of Applied Sciences & Research and Development Cell, Parul University, Vadodara, Gujarat, India
[c]School of Pharmaceutical Sciences, Lovely Professional University, Phagwara, Punjab, India
*Corresponding author. e-mail address: prabhakar.iitm@gmail.com

Contents

Advances in Immunology, Volume 165
ISSN 0065-2776, https://doi.org/10.1016/bs.ai.2024.10.010

Abstract

Malignant melanoma is one of the most aggressive forms of cancer and a leading cause of death from skin tumors. With the rising incidence of melanoma diagnoses, there is an urgent need to develop effective treatments. Among the most modern approaches are cancer vaccines, which aim to enhance cell-mediated immunity. Recently, mRNA-based cancer vaccines have gained significant attention due to their rapid production, low manufacturing costs, and ability to induce both humoral and cellular immune responses. These vaccines hold great potential in melanoma treatment, yet their application faces several challenges, including mRNA stabilization, delivery methods, and tumor heterogeneity. The recent success of mRNA vaccines in combating COVID-19 has renewed interest in their potential for cancer immunotherapy. In particular, mRNA cancer vaccines offer high specificity and better efficacy compared to traditional treatments. They can target tumor-specific neoantigens, prompting a robust immune response. This chapter reviews the mechanism of action of mRNA vaccines, advancements in adjuvant identification, and innovations in delivery systems such as lipid nanoparticles. It also discusses ongoing clinical trials evaluating the efficacy of mRNA-based vaccines in melanoma, highlighting promising early-phase results. Despite their potential, the development of mRNA cancer vaccines faces significant obstacles. Tumor heterogeneity, immunosuppressive tumor microenvironments, and practical issues like vaccine administration and clinical evaluation methods are major barriers to success. By addressing these challenges and advancing innovations, mRNA cancer vaccines hold promise for transforming melanoma treatment. A careful balance between the opportunities and challenges will be key to unlocking the full potential of mRNA vaccines in cancer immunotherapy.

1. Introduction

Cancer is a severe and complex disease that poses significant health challenges globally, resulting in high morbidity and mortality. Melanoma, a cancer originating from the melanocytes, is among the most aggressive types of skin cancer, characterized by a low survival rate. In the United States, the estimated incidence in 2024 reached approximately 2001,140 + new cases, with around 611,720 + deaths, a figure that continues to rise (American Cancer Society Cancer Facts & Statistics, 2024). A considerable number of cancers are caused by somatic mutations—changes in the DNA of cells that accumulate due to factors like exposure to carcinogens, genetic predisposition, and environmental influences. These mutations lead to the production of abnormal proteins, some of which are unique to cancer cells and not found in normal cells. These abnormal proteins, also known as neoantigens, are recognized as foreign by the immune system (Xie et al., 2023). Most neoantigens are unique to an individual patient, though some are shared among many patients due to common mutations in key proteins, such as p53 and KRAS (Zhang et al., 2021). Targeting these shared neoantigens offers the potential for broader and more affordable therapeutic interventions. In a healthy state, the immune system effectively eliminates such foreign entities, including abnormal cells like cancer cells. However, cancer cells often develop mechanisms to evade immune recognition and destruction. This is where immunotherapy has proven to be a breakthrough, revolutionizing cancer treatment by harnessing the immune system to target cancer cells (Bidram et al., 2021). Immunotherapy has shown remarkable results, especially in cases where traditional treatments like chemotherapy or radiation therapy have been ineffective. It has led to prolonged survival and even complete remission in some patients, offering new hope in cancer treatment.

One of the most notable immunotherapy strategies is immune checkpoint blockade. Immune checkpoint molecules help maintain immune balance and prevent excessive activation, but cancer cells can exploit these molecules to evade immune attacks. Drugs known as immune checkpoint inhibitors (ICIs) block these inhibitory signals, unleashing the immune system to recognize and destroy cancer cells (Lao et al., 2022). Another immunotherapy approach is adoptive cell therapy (ACT), where, for example, chimeric antigen receptor T cells (CAR-T cells) are engineered to specifically target cancer cells, showing great success in treating certain types of blood cancers (Mohanty et al., 2019). Despite these advancements, the development of effective cancer vaccines has lagged behind. Provenge, a tumor vaccine approved by the FDA in 2010 for treating castration-resistant prostate cancer, was initially promising but ultimately faded from use due to high costs and limited efficacy (He et al., 2023). Nevertheless, the maturity of mRNA technology offers new hope for cancer vaccines, particularly in addressing the limitations faced by earlier vaccine approaches. The global expansion of mRNA technology, propelled by its success in the COVID-19 pandemic, has accelerated research in cancer vaccines. mRNA vaccines have emerged as a promising platform, offering several advantages over conventional vaccines, such as cost-effective manufacturing, safe administration, and rapid development (Fig. 1). One of the key advantages of mRNA vaccines is their ability to encode tumor-specific antigens, leading to the activation of immune responses against cancer cells. Compared to traditional vaccines, mRNA vaccines can induce a strong immune response, particularly by eliciting $CD8^+$ T-cell activity, which plays a critical role in eradicating tumors (Miao et al., 2021).

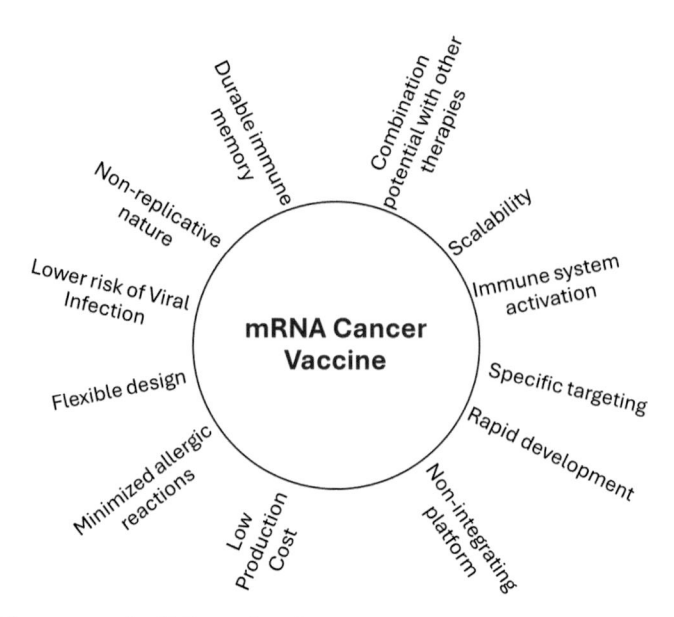

Fig. 1 Advantages of mRNA vaccines in cancer management.

mRNA cancer vaccines work by introducing single-stranded molecules that encode neoantigen proteins. These mRNA molecules are delivered into the cytoplasm of antigen-presenting cells, such as dendritic cells (DCs), where they are translated into neoantigens (Beck et al., 2021). The neoantigens stimulate DCs through Toll-like receptors, promoting a robust immune response. The mRNA vaccines also induce a strong type I interferon response, enhancing their efficacy in activating T-cells that target and destroy cancer cells. However, mRNA vaccines are not without challenges. Their instability and inefficient in vivo delivery limit their widespread application. Researchers are actively working on modifications to improve mRNA structure and formulation, such as codon optimization, nucleotide modification, and the use of lipid nanoparticles (LNPs) to enhance stability and efficacy. The success of mRNA vaccines in the COVID-19 pandemic, particularly with vaccines like mRNA-1273 and BNT162b2, has reignited interest in mRNA-based cancer vaccines. These vaccines showed the ability to stimulate a robust immune response by encoding viral spike proteins, paving the way for similar strategies in cancer treatment (Li et al., 2024). The simplicity and safety profile of mRNA vaccines, coupled with their rapid development potential, make them a promising platform for cancer immunotherapy.

Melanoma, one of the most aggressive forms of skin cancer, presents a promising target for mRNA cancer vaccines due to its high mutation burden. Immunotherapies like ipilimumab, nivolumab, and pembrolizumab have already shown efficacy in treating advanced melanoma by enhancing the immune system's ability to target cancer cells. mRNA cancer vaccines hold further potential in melanoma treatment by leveraging the tumor's high mutation rate to generate a wide array of neoantigens for vaccine formulation. Unlike traditional cancer treatments such as chemotherapy, which can damage healthy cells, immunotherapies are designed to target cancer cells specifically (Bidram et al., 2021). This precision reduces side effects and improves treatment outcomes. Cancer vaccines aim to induce a specific immune response by using tumor antigens to trigger an antitumor response, leading to tumor removal. Various types of cancer vaccines are being explored, including those based on dendritic cells, recombinant viruses, DNA, and mRNA. mRNA vaccines, in particular, stand out due to their versatility and rapid development capabilities. They offer a superior safety profile compared to other vaccine platforms, such as viral vectors, as they only contain the elements necessary for protein expression. mRNA vaccines can be designed to deliver monoclonal antibodies, induce the death of cancer cells, modulate the tumor microenvironment, and generate cancer-specific T cells (Bidram et al., 2021).

Despite the potential of mRNA vaccines, there are still significant challenges to overcome. The immunosuppressive tumor microenvironment and mechanisms of immune evasion by cancer cells represent major hurdles in the development of effective cancer vaccines. Researchers are actively exploring strategies to improve vaccine efficacy, such as enhancing the stability and delivery of mRNA molecules and optimizing vaccine formulations to boost immune responses. mRNA cancer vaccines represent a promising frontier in cancer immunotherapy (Li et al., 2022). The success of mRNA technology in the COVID-19 pandemic has accelerated research in this field, offering new hope for effective cancer treatments. While challenges remain, ongoing advancements in mRNA vaccine development hold the potential to revolutionize cancer treatment, providing a powerful tool in the fight against this devastating disease.

2. Melanoma: biology and immunological landscape

Melanoma is a malignant tumor that arises from melanocytes, the pigment-producing cells of the skin. It is one of the most aggressive forms of skin cancer and accounts for a significant proportion of skin cancer-related mortality. The molecular mechanisms and genetic mutations that drive melanoma development and progression are complex and involve multiple pathways. One of the critical genetic alterations in melanoma is the mutation of the BRAF gene, particularly the V600E mutation, which is present in about 40–60 % of melanomas. The BRAF gene encodes a serine/threonine-protein kinase involved in the MAPK/ERK signaling pathway, which regulates cell growth and division. The V600E mutation leads to the constitutive activation of BRAF, promoting uncontrolled cell proliferation and tumorigenesis. This discovery has paved the way for targeted therapies such as BRAF inhibitors (e.g., vemurafenib, dabrafenib), which specifically inhibit the mutant BRAF protein, leading to tumor regression in many patients (Bahar et al., 2023).

Another critical genetic alteration in melanoma is the mutation in the NRAS gene, occurring in approximately 15–20 % of melanomas. NRAS mutations also activate the MAPK pathway, contributing to tumor growth. Unlike BRAF-mutant melanomas, NRAS-mutant melanomas do not respond well to BRAF inhibitors, and effective targeted therapies for NRAS mutations are still being developed (Haanen and Robert, 2015; Lao et al., 2022). The TP53 gene, which encodes the tumor suppressor protein p53, is also frequently mutated in melanoma. p53 plays a crucial role in DNA repair, apoptosis, and cell cycle regulation. Loss of p53 function allows melanoma cells to evade apoptosis and continue proliferating despite accumulating DNA damage. Other tumor suppressor genes implicated in melanoma include CDKN2A, which encodes two proteins, p16^INK4a^ and p14^ARF^, involved in cell cycle regulation. Mutations in CDKN2A are found in familial melanoma cases and in a subset of sporadic melanomas, contributing to cell cycle dysregulation and tumorigenesis. In addition to these well-known mutations, melanoma can exhibit alterations in various other genes, including **PTEN**, which negatively regulates the PI3K/AKT pathway, and **KIT**, a receptor tyrosine kinase mutated in some mucosal and acral melanomas. The genetic heterogeneity of melanoma contributes to its aggressive nature and complicates treatment strategies.

2.1 Immune evasion strategies of melanoma cells

Melanoma is a highly immunogenic tumor, meaning that it can provoke an immune response. However, melanoma cells have developed several immune evasion strategies that allow them to avoid detection and destruction by the immune system. These strategies include alterations in antigen presentation, immune checkpoint modulation, and the creation of an immunosuppressive tumor microenvironment. One of the primary mechanisms by which melanoma cells evade the immune system is through the downregulation of major histocompatibility complex (MHC) molecules. MHC molecules are essential for presenting tumor antigens to T cells, which are critical for initiating an immune response. By reducing MHC expression, melanoma cells decrease the likelihood of being recognized by cytotoxic T lymphocytes (CTLs), which are responsible for killing tumor cells (Fig. 2). Some melanomas also lose the expression of tumor-associated antigens (TAAs) or tumor-specific antigens (TSAs), further reducing their immunogenicity (Haanen and Robert, 2015; Lao et al., 2022). Melanoma cells also exploit immune checkpoint pathways to suppress immune responses. Immune checkpoints are regulatory molecules that maintain immune homeostasis and prevent excessive immune activation. Two of the most well-known immune checkpoint molecules are programmed cell death protein 1 (PD-1) and cytotoxic T-lymphocyte-associated protein 4 (CTLA-4) (Cui et al., 2024). PD-1 is expressed on activated T cells, and its ligands, PD-L1 and PD-L2, are often upregulated on melanoma cells and other cells within the tumor microenvironment. The interaction between PD-1 and PD-L1 inhibits T cell function, allowing melanoma cells to evade immune

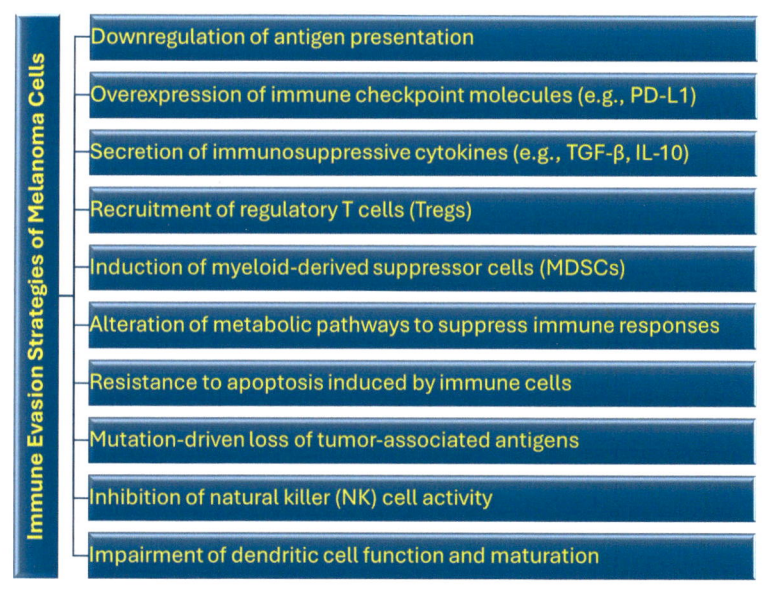

Fig. 2 Immune evasion strategies of melanoma cells.

surveillance. Similarly, CTLA-4 competes with the costimulatory molecule CD28 for binding to B7 ligands on antigen-presenting cells, leading to decreased T cell activation (Song et al., 2018).

The tumor microenvironment (TME) of melanoma is another critical factor in immune evasion. The TME is composed of various immune cells, stromal cells, and extracellular matrix components that can either promote or inhibit tumor growth. Melanoma cells often create an immunosuppressive TME by recruiting regulatory T cells (Tregs) and myeloid-derived suppressor cells (MDSCs), which inhibit the activity of effector T cells (Chakraborty et al., 2024). Additionally, melanoma cells secrete immunosuppressive cytokines, such as transforming growth factor-beta (TGF-β) and interleukin-10 (IL-10), which further dampen the immune response. The process of T cell exhaustion also plays a role in immune evasion. Chronic exposure to tumor antigens can lead to the functional impairment of T cells, characterized by the upregulation of inhibitory receptors such as PD-1, CTLA-4, TIM-3, and LAG-3. Exhausted T cells are less effective at killing melanoma cells, allowing the tumor to progress (Cui et al., 2024; Umansky and Sevko, 2013).

2.2 Current immunotherapies in melanoma

The advent of immunotherapy has revolutionized the treatment of melanoma, particularly for patients with advanced or metastatic disease. Immunotherapies aim to harness the power of the immune system to recognize and eliminate melanoma cells, and several approaches have been developed, including checkpoint inhibitors, adoptive cell therapy, and cancer vaccines (Fig. 3). Checkpoint inhibitors are the most successful class of immunotherapies in melanoma treatment. As mentioned earlier, melanoma cells exploit immune checkpoint pathways to evade immune detection. Blocking these pathways with immune checkpoint inhibitors (ICIs) can restore T cell function and enhance the immune response against melanoma (Haanen and Robert, 2015; Lao et al., 2022). The first immune checkpoint inhibitor approved for melanoma was ipilimumab, an anti-CTLA-4 monoclonal antibody. Ipilimumab works by blocking CTLA-4, thereby promoting T cell activation and proliferation. Clinical trials have shown that ipilimumab can improve overall survival in patients with advanced melanoma, although it is associated with significant immune-related adverse events due to its broad activation of the immune system. Following the success of ipilimumab, the focus shifted to the PD-1/PD-L1 pathway. Nivolumab and pembrolizumab, both anti-PD-1 antibodies,

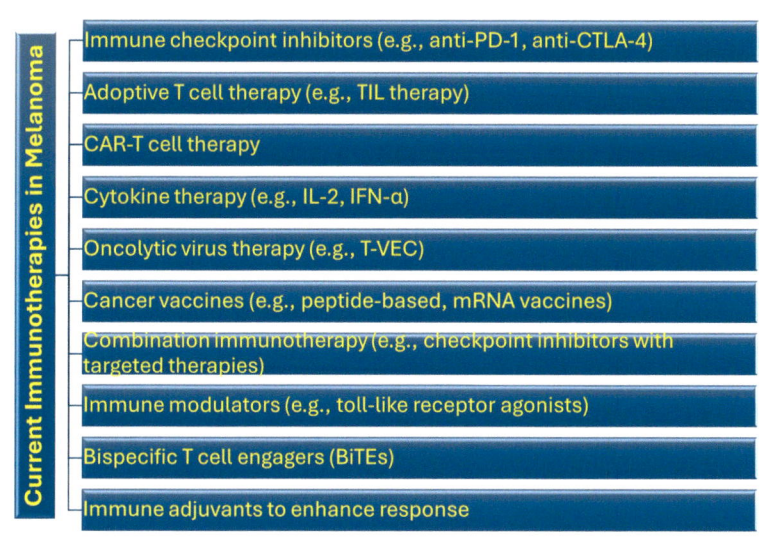

Fig. 3 Overview of current immunotherapies in melanoma. The figure illustrates various therapeutic strategies including immune checkpoint inhibitors (e.g., anti-PD-1, anti-CTLA-4), adoptive T cell therapy (e.g., TIL therapy), CAR-T cell therapy, cytokine therapy (e.g., IL-2, IFN-α), oncolytic virus therapy (e.g., T-VEC), cancer vaccines (e.g., peptide-based, mRNA vaccines), combination immunotherapies, immune modulators (e.g., toll-like receptor agonists), bispecific T cell engagers (BiTEs), and immune adjuvants. These therapies represent cutting-edge approaches to harness the immune system for effective melanoma treatment.

were approved for the treatment of advanced melanoma. These drugs block the interaction between PD-1 on T cells and PD-L1 on tumor cells, restoring T cell activity and promoting tumor destruction. Compared to ipilimumab, anti-PD-1 therapies have shown higher response rates and are generally better tolerated (Cui et al., 2024; Rojas et al., 2023). The combination of nivolumab and ipilimumab has also been approved for melanoma and has demonstrated improved efficacy compared to either drug alone, although the combination is associated with increased toxicity.

Despite the success of checkpoint inhibitors, not all patients respond to these therapies. About 20–30 % of melanoma patients do not benefit from ICIs, highlighting the need for additional therapeutic strategies. Adoptive cell therapy (ACT) is another promising approach in melanoma treatment. ACT involves the isolation and expansion of tumor-infiltrating lympho-cytes (TILs) from a patient's tumor, followed by reinfusion into the patient after lymphodepletion (Sayour et al., 2024). The expanded TILs are enriched for melanoma-specific T cells, which can directly attack tumor cells. ACT has shown impressive results in some melanoma patients, particularly those who are refractory to other treatments. However, the therapy is labor-intensive, costly, and only available at specialized centers. A specific form of ACT, chimeric antigen receptor (CAR) T-cell therapy, has also been explored in melanoma, though it has had more success in hematological malignancies than in solid tumors (Mohanty et al., 2019; Sayour et al., 2024). CAR-T cells are genetically engineered to express receptors that target specific antigens on tumor cells, but challenges such as the immunosuppressive TME have limited their effectiveness in melanoma. Cancer vaccines represent another approach to immunotherapy, aiming to stimulate the immune system to recognize and destroy melanoma cells. Melanoma, with its high mutation burden, presents many neoantigens that could serve as targets for vaccination. However, despite preclinical promise, cancer vaccines have not yet demonstrated significant clinical efficacy in melanoma, likely due to the immunosuppressive TME and the development of immune resistance mechanisms by the tumor. Advances in mRNA vaccine technology, as demonstrated during the COVID-19 pandemic, offer new hope for developing effective cancer vaccines in melanoma, as mRNA vaccines are highly immunogenic and can be rapidly designed to target specific tumor antigens.

Melanoma is a formidable cancer characterized by its aggressive nature and ability to evade immune surveillance. Its molecular mechanisms involve key mutations in pathways such as MAPK and PI3K, which drive uncontrolled cell growth and survival (Shirley et al., 2024). Melanoma cells have evolved multiple strategies to evade the immune system, including the downregulation of antigen presentation, exploitation of immune checkpoint pathways, and the creation of an immunosuppressive tumor microenvironment. Immunotherapy has transformed the treatment landscape for melanoma, with immune checkpoint inhibitors such as anti-CTLA-4 and anti-PD-1 antibodies leading the charge. These therapies have improved survival outcomes for many patients, though challenges such as resistance and toxicity remain. Adoptive cell therapies and cancer vaccines represent additional promising strategies, but further research is needed to overcome the hurdles of immune evasion and the immunosuppressive tumor environment. The future of melanoma treatment lies in a deeper understanding of its biology and immunological landscape, coupled with the continued development of innovative immunotherapies. By harnessing the full potential of the immune system, there is hope for more durable and effective treatments for melanoma patients.

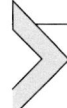

3. Principles of mRNA-based vaccines

3.1 History and evolution of mRNA vaccines

The concept of using messenger RNA (mRNA) as a platform for vaccines has evolved over the past several decades, culminating in the rapid development and deployment of mRNA vaccines during the COVID-19 pandemic. The story of mRNA vaccines is one of persistence, innovation, and the harnessing of fundamental biological processes to create a new generation of vaccines. The idea of using mRNA as a therapeutic tool was first proposed in the early 1990s. Katalin Karikó and Drew Weissman made seminal contributions to the field by overcoming a critical barrier: the high immunogenicity and instability of synthetic mRNA (Cui et al., 2024). Early attempts to use mRNA for therapeutic purposes were hampered by the fact that exogenous, or foreign, mRNA triggered strong immune responses, leading to rapid degradation of the mRNA before it could be translated into the desired protein. This posed a significant challenge to the development of mRNA as a vaccine platform. In the early 2000s, Karikó and Weissman discovered that modifying the nucleosides within the mRNA sequence reduced its recognition by the immune system, thus preventing its rapid degradation and allowing the mRNA to remain stable long enough to be translated into protein. This breakthrough was pivotal in making mRNA a feasible platform for vaccine development (Deng et al., 2022; Le et al., 2010). The introduction of modified nucleosides, such as pseudouridine, and improvements in delivery systems, such as LNPs, helped stabilize mRNA and ensure its efficient delivery into cells. The use of mRNA in vaccines gained significant attention during the COVID-19 pandemic. Within months of the identification of the SARS-CoV-2 virus, Pfizer-BioNTech and Moderna developed mRNA vaccines that received emergency use authorization. These vaccines demonstrated high efficacy in preventing severe illness and death from COVID-19, marking the first widespread clinical success of mRNA vaccines and setting the stage for future applications, including cancer immunotherapy.

3.2 Mechanism of action: encoding tumor antigens and immune activation

The mechanism of action of mRNA vaccines is fundamentally based on the central dogma of molecular biology: the process by which genetic information in DNA is transcribed into RNA, which is then translated into proteins. In the context of mRNA vaccines, synthetic mRNA is designed to encode a specific protein, which could be a viral antigen, bacterial protein, or TAA in cancer immunotherapy. Once the mRNA is delivered into cells, it is translated into the target protein, which then stimulates an immune response.

i. **mRNA Encoding Tumor Antigens:** For cancer immunotherapy, mRNA vaccines are designed to encode tumor antigens, which are proteins specifically expressed or overexpressed on the surface of cancer cells. These antigens can be TSAs or TAAs. TSAs are unique to cancer cells and arise from mutations or alterations in normal cellular proteins, while TAAs are expressed at higher levels in tumor cells but may also be found in normal tissues. In an mRNA cancer vaccine, once the synthetic mRNA encoding the tumor antigen is introduced into the body (usually through intramuscular or subcutaneous injection), the mRNA is taken up by DCs or other antigen–presenting cells (APCs). Inside the APCs, the mRNA is translated into the corresponding tumor antigen (Deng et al., 2022; Le et al., 2010). These newly synthesized antigens are then processed and presented on the cell surface in the context of MHC molecules (Carreno et al., 2015). The MHC class I pathway is responsible for presenting endogenous antigens, including those synthesized from the mRNA vaccine, to $CD8^+$ cytotoxic T cells. This leads to the activation of CD8 + T cells, which then recognize and kill tumor cells expressing the same antigen. The MHC class II pathway, on the other hand, presents antigens to $CD4^+$ helper T cells, which play a supportive role in enhancing the immune response by activating B cells and further stimulating $CD8^+$ T cells. In this way, mRNA vaccines aim to generate a strong and specific cytotoxic T–cell response, capable of targeting and eliminating cancer cells. Additionally, mRNA vaccines can encode multiple tumor antigens simultaneously, which helps to overcome the issue of tumor heterogeneity, where different tumor cells express different antigens.

ii. **Immune Activation:** Beyond encoding the antigen, mRNA itself can act as an immune stimulant, further boosting the immune response. The immune system has evolved to recognize foreign RNA as a potential indicator of viral infection. This recognition is mediated by pattern recognition receptors (PRRs), such as toll–like receptors (TLRs), RIG-I–like receptors (RLRs), and NOD–like receptors (NLRs), which detect the presence of foreign RNA and trigger innate immune responses. When mRNA vaccines are administered, the PRRs in immune cells detect the exogenous mRNA, leading to the production of type I interferons (IFNs) and other pro-inflammatory cytokines. These cytokines act as danger signals, recruiting and activating additional immune cells, including dendritic cells, macrophages, and natural killer (NK) cells, to the site of vaccination. This innate immune activation helps to amplify the subsequent adaptive immune response, including the generation of antigen-specific T cells and antibodies. The immune stimulatory properties of mRNA are a double-edged sword, as excessive activation of the innate immune system can lead to inflammation and adverse effects. This is why the development of mRNA vaccines has required careful optimization of the mRNA structure to balance immune activation with the need for antigen expression. The use of nucleoside modifications, as mentioned earlier, has been crucial in reducing the innate immune response to mRNA, ensuring that the vaccine can effectively trigger adaptive immunity without causing excessive inflammation.

3.3 Comparison with traditional vaccine platforms

mRNA vaccines represent a significant departure from traditional vaccine platforms, such as live-attenuated vaccines, inactivated vaccines, and subunit or peptide vaccines (Fig. 4). Each of these platforms has advantages and limitations, and understanding how mRNA vaccines compare to them provides insight into the unique benefits and challenges of this new technology.

i. **Live-Attenuated Vaccines:** Live-attenuated vaccines are made from viruses or bacteria that have been weakened so that they cannot cause disease but still replicate in the body and stimulate an immune response. Examples of live-attenuated vaccines include the measles, mumps, and rubella (MMR) vaccine and the yellow fever vaccine (Deng et al., 2022; Le et al., 2010).

Advantages:
- These vaccines generate strong and long-lasting immune responses, often mimicking natural infection.
- They induce both humoral (antibody-mediated) and cellular (T-cell-mediated) immunity.

Disadvantages:
- Live-attenuated vaccines can pose risks for individuals with compromised immune systems, as the weakened pathogen can sometimes regain virulence.

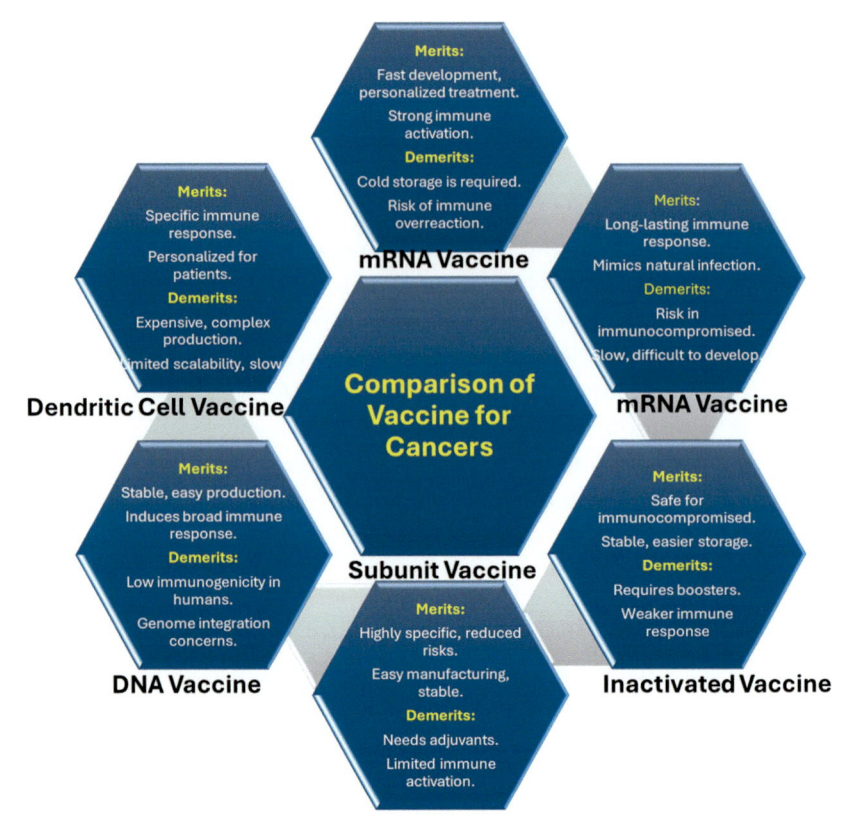

Fig. 4 Comparative overview of cancer vaccine platforms. The figure highlights the key merits and demerits of various cancer vaccine types.

- The development process is lengthy and complex, requiring careful attenuation of the pathogen to ensure safety.

Comparison to mRNA Vaccines:

- Unlike live-attenuated vaccines, mRNA vaccines do not contain any live pathogen, eliminating the risk of causing disease or reversion to a virulent form.
- mRNA vaccines can be developed much more rapidly, as they only require the genetic sequence of the pathogen or antigen of interest, making them well-suited for responding to emerging infectious diseases.
- However, the durability of immune responses generated by mRNA vaccines may not be as long-lasting as those produced by live-attenuated vaccines, necessitating booster doses in some cases.

i. Inactivated Vaccines: Inactivated vaccines contain viruses or bacteria that have been killed or inactivated so that they can no longer replicate or cause disease. Examples include the polio (IPV) vaccine and the hepatitis A vaccine (Deng et al., 2022; Le et al., 2010).

Advantages:

- These vaccines are generally very safe, as the pathogen is completely inactivated.
- They are suitable for individuals with weakened immune systems.

Disadvantages:

- Inactivated vaccines tend to induce weaker immune responses compared to live-attenuated vaccines and often require multiple doses or booster shots.
- They primarily stimulate humoral immunity, with limited activation of cellular immunity.

Comparison to mRNA Vaccines:

- Like inactivated vaccines, mRNA vaccines are non-infectious and cannot cause disease.
- However, mRNA vaccines have the advantage of inducing both humoral and cellular immune responses, making them more versatile in targeting a wider range of pathogens, including viruses and tumors.
- Additionally, mRNA vaccines can be rapidly produced and adapted, whereas the production of inactivated vaccines involves the labor-intensive process of growing and inactivating the pathogen.

i. Subunit and Peptide Vaccines: Subunit vaccines contain only specific proteins or peptides from the pathogen, rather than the whole organism. Examples include the hepatitis B vaccine and the human papillomavirus (HPV) vaccine (Deng et al., 2022; Le et al., 2010).

Advantages:

- These vaccines are very safe, as they contain no live pathogen and only a small portion of the antigen.
- They are often well-tolerated with minimal side effects.

Disadvantages:

- Subunit vaccines tend to elicit weaker immune responses and often require the use of **adjuvants** (substances that enhance the immune response).
- Multiple doses or boosters are often required to achieve protective immunity.

Comparison to mRNA Vaccines:

- mRNA vaccines offer several advantages over subunit vaccines, including the ability to encode multiple antigens simultaneously, thus targeting multiple aspects of a pathogen or cancer.

- mRNA vaccines can also stimulate stronger immune responses because the antigen is produced endogenously within cells, more closely resembling natural infection or tumor antigen expression.

i. **DNA Vaccines:** DNA vaccines are similar to mRNA vaccines in that they deliver genetic material encoding the antigen, but they use **plasmid DNA** rather than mRNA. The DNA is delivered into cells, where it is transcribed into mRNA and then translated into the target protein (Deng et al., 2022; Le et al., 2010).

Advantages:
- DNA vaccines are stable and easy to produce, with a relatively long shelf life compared to mRNA vaccines.
- They can elicit both humoral and cellular immune responses.

Disadvantages:
i. DNA vaccines face challenges in efficient delivery to cells, as the DNA must enter the cell nucleus to be transcribed, which requires more complex delivery methods.
ii. DNA vaccines may carry the risk of integration into the host genome, although this risk is considered low.

Comparison to mRNA Vaccines:
- mRNA vaccines have the advantage of not needing to enter the cell nucleus, as the mRNA is directly translated in the cytoplasm. This simplifies the delivery process and reduces potential safety concerns associated with genome integration.
- mRNA vaccines have a faster onset of action because they bypass the transcription step required for DNA vaccines.

i. **Dendritic Cell Vaccine for Cancer:** Dendritic cell vaccines are a form of cancer immunotherapy that harness the body's immune system by using activated dendritic cells to present tumor antigens to T cells. This targeted approach aims to stimulate a robust immune response specifically against cancer cells (Perez and De Palma, 2019).
  - **Advantages:**
    - o Dendritic cells present tumor antigens directly to T cells, leading to a highly targeted immune reaction.
    - o Custom-made using patient-specific tumor antigens for personalized therapy.
  - **Disadvantages:**
    - o Requires extraction, manipulation, and reinfusion of patient cells, leading to high costs and longer preparation times.

o Difficult to mass-produce and administer compared to other vaccine platforms.

Comparison to mRNA Vaccine:

- Higher specificity in activating T cells directly with tumor antigens.
- Better personalized targeting as dendritic cells are custom-tailored for individual patients.
- Slower development and manufacturing, while mRNA vaccines are faster and easier to produce.
- More expensive and labor-intensive, whereas mRNA vaccines offer easier scalability and lower production costs.

mRNA-based vaccines represent a transformative platform in vaccinology, offering rapid development, flexible design, and potent immune responses. Their ability to encode tumor antigens and stimulate both innate and adaptive immunity has opened new avenues for cancer immunotherapy. While mRNA vaccines have shown remarkable success in infectious disease settings, such as COVID-19, their potential for targeting cancers and other diseases is only beginning to be realized. The comparison with traditional vaccine platforms underscores the unique advantages of mRNA vaccines, particularly their safety profile, adaptability, and ability to elicit robust cellular immunity. As research into mRNA vaccines continues, they are poised to play a central role in the future of personalized medicine and cancer treatment.

4. mRNA vaccine development for melanoma

Melanoma, a malignant tumor originating from melanocytes, is one of the most aggressive forms of skin cancer. The incidence of melanoma has been rising globally, with a significant challenge posed by its ability to metastasize and develop resistance to conventional therapies. Traditional treatment modalities, including surgery, chemotherapy, and radiation, have limitations in terms of efficacy and side effects. As a result, there is a growing interest in novel therapeutic approaches, including mRNA-based vaccines, which have shown promise in stimulating robust immune responses against melanoma. This article will explore the selection of melanoma antigens for mRNA vaccines, the design and optimization of mRNA constructs, and the various delivery platforms, including lipid nanoparticles and dendritic cell vaccines.

4.1 Selection of melanoma antigens for mRNA vaccines

The selection of appropriate melanoma antigens is crucial for the efficacy of mRNA vaccines. Melanoma cells express a variety of antigens that can be targeted to stimulate an immune response. These antigens can be broadly categorized into two main types: TAAs and TSAs.

i. ***Tumor-Associated Antigens (TAAs):*** TAAs are proteins that are over-expressed or aberrantly expressed in tumor cells compared to normal cells. While these antigens can be found in normal tissues, they are often present at much higher levels in melanoma. Common TAAs associated with melanoma include:

- **Tyrosinase**: An enzyme involved in melanin biosynthesis, tyrosinase is a well-studied TAA that has been targeted in various melanoma vaccine trials.
- **Melan-A/MART-1**: This is another melanocyte differentiation antigen that is frequently overexpressed in melanoma and serves as a target for T cell-mediated responses (Rojas et al., 2023; Xie et al., 2023).
- **gp100**: A glycoprotein involved in the immune response, gp100 is another promising target for melanoma vaccines due to its over-expression in melanoma cells.

  While TAAs present a broader target pool, they can also lead to autoimmunity since they are present in normal tissues.

ii. **Tumor-Specific Antigens (TSAs):** TSAs are unique to cancer cells and arise from mutations that occur during tumorigenesis. Because these antigens are not present in normal cells, TSAs offer the potential for highly specific targeting, minimizing the risk of autoimmune responses. Examples of TSAs in melanoma include:

- **BRAF V600E:** A common mutation in melanoma, BRAF V600E produces a mutated protein that can be targeted by immune cells.
- **NRAS mutations:** Similar to BRAF, NRAS mutations lead to the production of altered proteins that can elicit a robust immune response.
- **Neoantigens:** These are derived from non-synonymous mutations in tumor cells. Neoantigens are highly immunogenic and can be specifically targeted by the immune system (Rojas et al., 2023; Xie et al., 2023).

The identification and validation of these antigens are critical steps in developing effective mRNA vaccines. Next-generation sequencing and bioinformatics tools are often employed to identify potential neoantigens from individual patients' tumor samples, allowing for the development of personalized mRNA vaccines that target specific mutations in a patient's melanoma.

4.2 Designing and optimizing mRNA constructs

Once suitable antigens have been selected, the next step is designing and optimizing the mRNA constructs that will encode these antigens. The design process involves several key considerations:

i. **mRNA Design:** The mRNA construct must include specific elements to ensure proper translation, stability, and immunogenicity (Cafri et al., 2020). Key components of an effective mRNA vaccine include:
- **5′ Cap Structure**: A modified 5′ cap structure enhances mRNA stability, facilitates ribosomal binding, and improves translation efficiency.
- **5′ UTR (Untranslated Region)**: The 5′ UTR can enhance translation initiation and stability. Elements such as the **Kozak sequence** can be incorporated to improve translation efficiency.
- **Coding Sequence**: The coding sequence should encode the target antigen, often optimized for codon usage to enhance expression in human cells. This may involve the use of **optimized codons** that are more frequently used in human genes.
- **3′ UTR**: The 3′ UTR can contribute to mRNA stability and regulation of translation. Polyadenylation (addition of a poly(A) tail) is also essential for mRNA stability and translation.
- **Nucleoside Modifications**: Incorporating modified nucleosides, such as **pseudouridine** or **5-methylcytidine**, can reduce innate immune recognition of mRNA, enhancing its stability and translational efficiency while decreasing the immunogenicity of the mRNA itself.

ii. **Incorporating Immunogenicity Enhancers:** To further enhance the immune response elicited by the mRNA vaccine, several strategies can be employed:
- **Signal Peptides**: Adding signal peptides to the mRNA constructs can enhance the secretion of the encoded protein, promoting more effective antigen presentation by dendritic cells and increasing the immune response.
- **Transmembrane Domains**: Including transmembrane domains can aid in the display of antigens on the surface of the presenting cells, facilitating recognition by T cells.

- **Adjuvants**: While mRNA vaccines can induce immune responses through their inherent immunogenic properties, co-formulation with adjuvants can further boost these responses. For example, including small molecules that activate TLRs can enhance the innate immune response.

iii. **Stability and Formulation:** Stability is a critical consideration for mRNA vaccines, as they can be prone to degradation in physiological conditions. Various formulations can be used to enhance stability, including:
  - **Lipid Nanoparticles (LNPs)**: LNPs protect the mRNA from degradation and facilitate its delivery into cells. They encapsulate mRNA and enable its transport through biological barriers (Eygeris et al., 2021; Żak and Zangi, 2021).
  - **Lyophilization**: Drying the mRNA vaccine formulation can improve shelf-life and stability during storage.

The choice of formulation can influence the pharmacokinetics and biodistribution of the mRNA vaccine, ultimately affecting its efficacy. Optimizing these factors is essential to ensure that the mRNA is effectively delivered to the target cells and translated into the desired antigen.

4.3 Delivery platforms: lipid nanoparticles and dendritic cell vaccines

The effective delivery of mRNA vaccines to target cells is crucial for their success. Two primary platforms for delivering mRNA vaccines are LNPs and dendritic cell vaccines. Each platform has its unique advantages and challenges.

a. *Lipid Nanoparticles (LNPs):* LNPs are lipid-based carriers that encapsulate mRNA molecules, facilitating their transport and delivery into cells. They are composed of various lipids, including cationic lipids, phospholipids, and cholesterol, which form a lipid bilayer that encapsulates the mRNA (Le et al., 2010).
  - **Mechanism of Action**: When injected into the body, LNPs interact with cell membranes, enabling the uptake of the mRNA through endocytosis. Once inside the cell, the mRNA is released from the LNPs and enters the cytoplasm, where it can be translated into protein (Eygeris et al., 2021; Żak and Zangi, 2021).

- **Advantages**:
  - **Efficacy**: LNPs significantly enhance the stability of mRNA and improve cellular uptake, leading to more efficient translation and higher antigen expression.
  - **Versatility**: LNPs can be tailored to optimize their physicochemical properties, allowing for customization based on the target cells and specific applications.
  - **Safety**: LNPs can minimize the risk of unintended immune responses, as they protect the mRNA from degradation and reduce exposure to the immune system.
- **Challenges**:
  - **Immunogenicity**: While LNPs can enhance mRNA stability and delivery, they may still trigger immune responses. Careful design is required to balance efficacy and tolerability.
  - **Manufacturing Complexity**: The production of LNPs can be complex and requires specialized techniques, which may pose challenges for large-scale manufacturing.
- b. *Dendritic Cell Vaccines:* DCs are key players in the immune response, acting as professional APCs that can activate T cells (Le et al., 2010). Dendritic cell vaccines are designed to deliver mRNA directly into DCs, either ex vivo or in vivo, to enhance their capacity to present tumor antigens to the immune system.
  - **Ex Vivo Dendritic Cell Vaccines**: In this approach, patient-derived dendritic cells are isolated from peripheral blood, transfected with mRNA encoding tumor antigens, and then reinfused into the patient. This method allows for the precise delivery of tumor antigens to the DCs, enhancing their ability to stimulate T cell responses.
  - **In Vivo Dendritic Cell Vaccines**: Alternatively, mRNA can be delivered using targeted delivery systems to ensure that it reaches dendritic cells directly within the body. This method is more challenging but offers the potential for a more physiologically relevant immune response.
- **Advantages**:
  - **Potent Immune Activation**: Dendritic cells are highly efficient at processing and presenting antigens, making them ideal candidates for enhancing the immune response to mRNA vaccines.
  - **Personalization**: Ex vivo DC vaccines can be tailored to the individual patient, allowing for the selection of specific antigens based on tumor profiling.

- **Challenges**:
- **Complexity**: The ex vivo approach requires a more complex manufacturing process and specialized facilities for isolating and culturing dendritic cells.
- **Cost**: The individualized nature of dendritic cell vaccines can make them more expensive compared to standard mRNA vaccines.

The development of mRNA vaccines for melanoma represents a promising frontier in cancer immunotherapy. By carefully selecting melanoma antigens, optimizing mRNA constructs, and utilizing effective delivery platforms, researchers are working to enhance the immunogenicity and efficacy of these vaccines. The ability to generate personalized mRNA vaccines targeting unique tumor antigens is particularly exciting, as it offers the potential for tailored therapies that improve patient outcomes. As the field continues to advance, the integration of mRNA vaccine technology into clinical practice may transform the landscape of melanoma treatment and pave the way for new therapeutic strategies for other cancers. The challenges of manufacturing, delivery, and immune modulation must be addressed to fully realize the potential of mRNA vaccines, but the progress made thus far is a testament to their promise in modern medicine.

5. Mechanism of action in mRNA cancer vaccines

The advent of mRNA vaccines has revolutionized the field of cancer immunotherapy, offering a novel approach to stimulating the immune system to recognize and destroy tumor cells. Unlike traditional vaccines, mRNA cancer vaccines work by encoding tumor-specific antigens, which are then translated into proteins within the body. These proteins serve as "flags" that alert the immune system to the presence of cancer cells. By harnessing the body's immune response, mRNA vaccines aim to eradicate cancer while minimizing off-target effects. This approach is particularly promising in the treatment of melanoma, a highly aggressive form of skin cancer with a high mutational burden (Wei and Hui, 2022). In this article, we will delve into the intricate mechanism of action of mRNA cancer vaccines, focusing on the translation of mRNA into tumor-specific antigens, the activation of CD4 + and CD8 + T cells, and the role of mRNA vaccines in breaking immune tolerance in melanoma.

5.1 Translation of mRNA into tumor-specific antigens

At the core of mRNA cancer vaccines is the delivery of messenger RNA (mRNA) encoding TSAs or TAAs. These antigens are proteins or peptides that are either uniquely expressed or overexpressed in cancer cells, making them ideal targets for immune-mediated destruction.

1. **mRNA Delivery and Uptake:** The first step in the mechanism of action of mRNA cancer vaccines involves the delivery of the mRNA into host cells, typically using LNPs or other delivery vehicles (Wei and Hui, 2022). LNPs encapsulate the mRNA, protecting it from degradation and facilitating its uptake by APCs, such as DCs. Upon administration, LNPs bind to the cell surface and are internalized via endocytosis. Once inside the cell, the mRNA is released from the endosome into the cytoplasm, where it can be translated into protein.

2. **Translation of mRNA into Antigen:** After entering the cytoplasm, the host cell's ribosomes bind to the mRNA and initiate translation. The mRNA contains specific coding sequences that instruct the ribosomes to synthesize the tumor-specific antigen (Braun and Wu, 2017). This process mimics the natural protein synthesis that occurs in cells, allowing the antigen to be produced endogenously.

   - **Antigen Processing**: The newly synthesized tumor antigen is then processed by the host cell's machinery. In most cases, the antigen undergoes proteasomal degradation, resulting in smaller peptide fragments. These peptides are then transported into the endoplasmic reticulum (ER) by the transporter associated with antigen processing (TAP).
   - **Antigen Presentation**: In the ER, the peptide fragments are loaded onto MHC molecules. MHC class I molecules present the antigens on the surface of the cell, where they can be recognized by $CD8^+$ T cells (Cui et al., 2024). If the mRNA vaccine is designed to elicit a $CD4^+$ T cell response, the antigen can also be processed via the endosomal pathway and presented on MHC class II molecules.

This antigen presentation is crucial for the subsequent activation of the immune system, as it allows T cells to recognize and target cells expressing the tumor-specific antigen.

5.2 Activation of the immune system

The central goal of mRNA cancer vaccines is to activate the immune system to mount a robust response against cancer cells. This involves the activation of both $CD4^+$ helper T cells and CD8 + cytotoxic T cells, which play complementary roles in mediating the anti-tumor immune response.

i. **CD8 + Cytotoxic T Cells:** $CD8^+$ T cells, also known as cytotoxic T lymphocytes (CTLs), are the primary effectors in eliminating cancer cells. The activation of $CD8^+$ T cells by mRNA vaccines follows several key steps:

- **Antigen Recognition:** Once the tumor-specific antigens are presented on MHC class I molecules on the surface of antigen-presenting cells, $CD8^+$ T cells recognize these antigens through their T cell receptor (TCR). The binding of the TCR to the antigen-MHC complex provides the first signal for T cell activation (Cui et al., 2024).

- **Co-stimulation:** T cell activation also requires a second signal, provided by co-stimulatory molecules on the surface of APCs. For example, the interaction between CD28 on the T cell and B7 molecules on the APC delivers a necessary co-stimulatory signal, ensuring full T cell activation.

- **T Cell Proliferation and Differentiation:** After receiving both the antigenic and co-stimulatory signals, $CD8^+$ T cells undergo clonal expansion, proliferating to produce a large pool of effector cells. These effector $CD8^+$ T cells differentiate into cytotoxic T lymphocytes, which are capable of directly killing cancer cells.

- **Cytotoxic Activity:** CTLs kill cancer cells by recognizing the tumor-specific antigens presented on MHC class I molecules. Upon recognition, CTLs release cytotoxic granules containing perforin and granzymes. Perforin forms pores in the membrane of the target cell, allowing granzymes to enter the cell and induce apoptosis (programmed cell death).

  By targeting cells that express tumor-specific antigens, $CD8^+$ T cells provide a precise and effective means of eradicating cancer cells while sparing healthy tissues.

ii. **$CD4^+$ Helper T Cells:** $CD4^+$ T cells, also known as helper T cells, play a crucial role in orchestrating the broader immune response. While $CD8^+$ T cells are directly involved in killing cancer cells, $CD4^+$ T cells provide essential support by activating other immune cells and enhancing the cytotoxic activity of $CD8^+$ T cells.

- **Antigen Recognition:** $CD4^+$ T cells recognize tumor-specific antigens presented on MHC class II molecules on the surface of

APCs. Similar to $CD8^+$ T cells, $CD4^+$ T cells require both an antigenic signal and a co-stimulatory signal for activation.

- **Helper Functions:** Once activated, $CD4^+$ T cells secrete cytokines, such as interleukin-2 (IL-2), interferon-gamma (IFN-γ), and tumor necrosis factor–alpha (TNF-α), which promote the activation and proliferation of $CD8^+$ T cells, B cells, and macrophages. These cytokines enhance the overall immune response, ensuring that the immune system can effectively target and destroy cancer cells.
- **Memory T Cells:** In addition to their helper functions, $CD4^+$ T cells can differentiate into memory T cells. These long-lived cells persist in the body after the initial immune response and provide lasting protection by rapidly responding to future encounters with the same tumor antigen.

By activating both $CD8^+$ and $CD4^+$ T cells, mRNA cancer vaccines generate a coordinated immune response that targets tumor cells while also establishing immune memory.

5.3 Role in breaking immune tolerance in melanoma

One of the major challenges in treating melanoma is the ability of tumor cells to evade immune detection and suppress the immune response. This phenomenon, known as immune tolerance, allows melanoma cells to proliferate and spread without being attacked by the immune system. mRNA cancer vaccines offer a promising strategy for breaking immune tolerance and restoring the immune system's ability to recognize and eliminate melanoma cells.

i. **Overcoming Immune Suppression:** Melanoma cells employ various mechanisms to suppress the immune response, including the expression of immune checkpoint molecules (e.g., PD-L1) and the recruitment of regulatory T cells (Tregs) and myeloid-derived suppressor cells (MDSCs). These mechanisms create an immunosuppressive microenvironment that inhibits the activity of effector T cells and allows melanoma cells to evade immune surveillance (Cui et al., 2024). mRNA cancer vaccines can help overcome these suppressive mechanisms by promoting a strong, antigen-specific immune response that overwhelms the tumor's immune evasion strategies. For example, by inducing the activation of large numbers of $CD8^+$ and $CD4^+$ T cells, mRNA vaccines can counteract the effects of immune checkpoint molecules and suppressive cells. Moreover, the inclusion of adjuvants in mRNA vaccine formulations can further enhance immune activation and reduce immune tolerance.

ii. **Inducing Tumor-Specific Immunity:** Melanoma is characterized by a high mutational burden, resulting in the expression of numerous neoantigens—tumor-specific antigens derived from somatic mutations. These neoantigens are not present in normal tissues and therefore represent ideal targets for immune-mediated destruction (Deng et al., 2022). mRNA cancer vaccines can be designed to encode these neoantigens, allowing the immune system to specifically target melanoma cells while sparing healthy cells. By focusing the immune response on these tumor-specific antigens, mRNA vaccines help break immune tolerance and direct the immune system's attention to the tumor.

- **Neoantigen Vaccines**: Personalized mRNA vaccines can be developed based on the unique mutational profile of an individual's tumor. By identifying and encoding neoantigens that are specific to the patient's melanoma, these vaccines can generate a highly personalized immune response that is tailored to the patient's specific tumor.

iii. **Enhancing Tumor Antigen Presentation:** Another key aspect of breaking immune tolerance involves enhancing the presentation of tumor antigens to the immune system. Melanoma cells often down-regulate MHC class I molecules, limiting their ability to present antigens to $CD8^+$ T cells. This impairs the immune system's ability to recognize and target melanoma cells (Deng et al., 2022). mRNA cancer vaccines address this issue by delivering tumor antigens directly to professional APCs, such as dendritic cells. These APCs process the antigens and present them on MHC class I and II molecules, effectively bypassing the tumor's ability to evade immune detection. By enhancing antigen presentation, mRNA vaccines restore the immune system's ability to recognize melanoma cells and initiate an effective immune response.

The mechanism of action of mRNA cancer vaccines involves a complex interplay of processes that culminate in the activation of a robust anti-tumor immune response. By delivering mRNA encoding tumor-specific antigens, these vaccines enable the translation of antigens within host cells, leading to their presentation on MHC molecules and subsequent activation of $CD8^+$ and $CD4^+$ T cells. The ability of mRNA vaccines to break immune tolerance in melanoma, through enhanced antigen presentation and immune activation, represents a significant advance in cancer immunotherapy. As research continues to optimize mRNA vaccine design, delivery, and efficacy, this technology holds great promise for transforming the treatment of melanoma and other cancers.

6. Clinical trials and efficacy

The development of mRNA-based cancer vaccines has created a new paradigm in cancer immunotherapy, offering a platform that can be rapidly developed, easily modified, and personalized for each patient. Over the past decade, mRNA vaccines have been the subject of numerous preclinical and clinical trials, especially in cancer treatment. Clinical trials are essential for determining mRNA vaccines' safety, efficacy, and potential in combating various malignancies. This article provides a detailed overview of completed and ongoing clinical trials involving mRNA cancer vaccines, showcases success stories and case studies that demonstrate their therapeutic potential, and discusses the limitations and challenges in clinical outcomes.

6.1 Overview of completed and ongoing clinical trials

The journey of mRNA cancer vaccines from preclinical development to human clinical trials has been marked by significant progress. Below, we highlight key completed and ongoing clinical trials in this domain.

1. **Early-Phase Clinical Trials (Phase I and II):** The first phase I and II trials for mRNA cancer vaccines focused on assessing their safety, immunogenicity, and preliminary efficacy in treating various cancers, including melanoma, non-small cell lung cancer (NSCLC), and prostate cancer. These early trials helped establish the foundational principles of mRNA vaccine delivery and immune activation.

   - **Melanoma Trials**: Melanoma has been one of the primary cancers for which mRNA vaccines have been tested. One of the earliest trials involved patients with advanced-stage melanoma who received a personalized mRNA vaccine encoding neoantigens unique to their tumor. This trial (NCT02035956), led by BioNTech, aimed to stimulate a potent immune response to melanoma-specific neoantigens and demonstrated promising results in terms of immunogenicity and clinical outcomes (Wang et al., 2023). The vaccine was well-tolerated and induced robust $CD8^+$ and $CD4^+$ T cell responses specific to the neoantigens.

- **Prostate Cancer Trials:** In a phase I trial (NCT03480152), an mRNA vaccine encoding prostate-specific antigen (PSA) was tested in patients with metastatic prostate cancer. The vaccine was delivered using dendritic cells as a carrier to enhance antigen presentation and immune activation (Wang et al., 2023). Although early results indicated some level of immunogenicity, the overall clinical benefits were modest, highlighting the need for further optimization.
- **Lung Cancer Trials:** NSCLC, a highly prevalent cancer with limited treatment options, has also been targeted by mRNA vaccines. A trial conducted by Moderna (NCT03313778) investigated mRNA-4157, an individualized mRNA cancer vaccine designed to target multiple neoantigens. The trial combined mRNA-4157 with pembrolizumab, an anti-PD-1 checkpoint inhibitor, to enhance immune activation (Wang et al., 2023). Early results showed that the vaccine was safe and well-tolerated, with some patients demonstrating an objective response to the treatment.

2. **Later–Phase Clinical Trials (Phase III):** As the early-phase trials demonstrated the safety and feasibility of mRNA vaccines, larger phase III trials were initiated to assess their efficacy in a broader patient population.

   - **Key Trials in Melanoma:** Moderna's mRNA-4157 vaccine entered a phase II clinical trial (NCT03897881) involving patients with high-risk resected melanoma. The trial evaluated the efficacy of combining mRNA-4157 with pembrolizumab as an adjuvant therapy to prevent melanoma recurrence (Rojas et al., 2023). Preliminary results have shown that the combination reduced the risk of recurrence and improved overall survival compared to pembrolizumab alone.
   - **Personalized Neoantigen Vaccines:** BioNTech's ongoing clinical trial (NCT03815058) involves individualized mRNA vaccines targeting neoantigens in patients with melanoma and NSCLC (Rojas et al., 2023). This phase II trial evaluates the efficacy of the vaccine in combination with anti-PD-1 therapy. Interim analyses have revealed promising immune responses, and several patients have shown durable clinical benefit, suggesting the potential of personalized mRNA vaccines in combination with immunotherapy.
   - **Pancreatic Cancer Trials:** Pancreatic cancer is notoriously difficult to treat, and recent trials have explored mRNA vaccines as a new avenue for therapy. In a phase II trial (NCT04161755), BioNTech is testing a personalized mRNA vaccine targeting neoantigens in

combination with checkpoint inhibitors (Rojas et al., 2023). While early results are pending, the trial represents a significant step toward expanding the use of mRNA vaccines in hard-to-treat cancers.

3. **Ongoing Trials in Other Cancers:** Ongoing clinical trials are exploring mRNA vaccines in a variety of cancers beyond melanoma and lung cancer. These trials seek to assess the broader applicability of mRNA vaccines across different tumor types.

- **Head and Neck Cancer**: Moderna is conducting a phase I trial (NCT03983954) of mRNA-5671, an mRNA vaccine targeting KRAS mutations in patients with head and neck squamous cell carcinoma. KRAS is a common driver mutation in many cancers, and this trial aims to evaluate whether targeting KRAS-mutant tumors with an mRNA vaccine can induce a strong immune response (Wei and Hui, 2022).
- **Colorectal Cancer**: Several trials are underway to test mRNA vaccines in colorectal cancer, including a phase II trial (NCT04486378) that combines a personalized mRNA vaccine with anti-PD-L1 therapy in patients with microsatellite instability-high (MSI-H) colorectal cancer (Wei and Hui, 2022). The goal is to determine whether mRNA vaccines can boost the efficacy of checkpoint inhibitors in this subset of patients.
- **Breast Cancer**: mRNA vaccines are being explored in HER2-positive breast cancer, where HER2-targeted mRNA vaccines are designed to elicit an immune response against the HER2 protein. A phase I trial (NCT02316457) is testing the safety and immunogenicity of a HER2 mRNA vaccine in patients with metastatic breast cancer, with early results showing promising immune activation.

6.2 Success stories and case studies

While mRNA cancer vaccines are still in the clinical development phase, there have been notable success stories and case studies that highlight their therapeutic potential.

i. **Neoantigen Vaccines in Melanoma:** In one of the most notable success stories, a personalized neoantigen mRNA vaccine developed by BioNTech was used to treat patients with metastatic melanoma. In this case, the vaccine was tailored to the unique mutational profile of each patient's tumor, encoding up to 20 neoantigens. The vaccine was administered in combination with pembrolizumab (Xie et al., 2023;

Zhang et al., 2021). Several patients experienced partial or complete tumor regression, and some had durable responses lasting more than two years. These results suggest that personalized mRNA vaccines have the potential to generate long-lasting anti-tumor immunity and improve clinical outcomes in melanoma patients.

ii. **Combination Therapies with Checkpoint Inhibitors:** Checkpoint inhibitors, such as anti-PD-1 and anti-CTLA-4 therapies, have transformed cancer treatment by blocking immune checkpoints that suppress T cell activation. When combined with mRNA vaccines, these therapies can further enhance the immune response against tumors. One success story involves a patient with advanced NSCLC who received an individualized mRNA vaccine targeting neoantigens along with pembrolizumab. The patient experienced a significant reduction in tumor size, and the disease remained stable for over a year. This case highlights the potential synergy between mRNA vaccines and checkpoint inhibitors in promoting durable anti-tumor responses.

iii. **Long-Term Immunity and Memory:** One of the unique advantages of mRNA vaccines is their ability to induce long-term immune memory. In a case study involving a patient with prostate cancer, an mRNA vaccine encoding prostate-specific antigen (PSA) was administered along with standard-of-care treatments. The patient demonstrated a sustained immune response against PSA, and follow-up assessments revealed that the vaccine had induced the formation of long-lasting memory T cells. This suggests that mRNA vaccines may not only provide immediate therapeutic benefits but also confer long-term protection against cancer recurrence.

6.3 Limitations and challenges in clinical outcomes

Despite the promising results from early-phase clinical trials and case studies, mRNA cancer vaccines face several limitations and challenges that must be addressed to achieve widespread clinical success (Liu et al., 2023; Sayour et al., 2024).

i. **Immunogenicity and Tumor Heterogeneity:** One of the key challenges in developing effective mRNA vaccines is the variability in immune responses among patients. While some patients mount robust immune responses to the mRNA vaccine, others may experience only weak or transient responses. This variability can be attributed to several factors, including the patient's immune status, the quality of antigen presentation, and the tumor's ability to evade immune detection.

- **Tumor Heterogeneity:** Tumor cells are genetically diverse, and this heterogeneity can make it difficult to target all tumor cells with a single mRNA vaccine. Some tumor cells may not express the target antigens, allowing them to escape immune recognition. To address this issue, personalized mRNA vaccines that target multiple neoantigens are being developed, but tumor heterogeneity remains a significant hurdle to achieving complete tumor eradication.
- **Delivery and Stability of mRNA Vaccines:** Efficient delivery of mRNA into target cells is critical for the success of mRNA vaccines. However, mRNA is inherently unstable and prone to degradation by nucleases in the body. To overcome this challenge, LNPs are commonly used to protect the mRNA and facilitate its uptake by antigen-presenting cells. While LNPs have shown promise in preclinical and early-phase clinical trials, there are still concerns regarding their stability, toxicity, and efficiency in delivering mRNA to the intended target cells.
- **Toxicity and Adverse Effects:** In some cases, LNPs have been associated with inflammatory responses and other adverse effects. Balancing the need for effective mRNA delivery with minimizing toxicity remains a key challenge in optimizing mRNA vaccine formulations.

ii. **Immunosuppressive Tumor Microenvironment:** The tumor microenvironment (TME) plays a crucial role in shaping the immune response to cancer. In many cancers, including melanoma, the TME is highly immunosuppressive, containing regulatory T cells (Tregs), myeloid-derived suppressor cells (MDSCs), and other factors that inhibit anti-tumor immune responses. This immunosuppressive environment can limit the efficacy of mRNA vaccines by preventing T cells from effectively attacking tumor cells.

- **Overcoming Immune Suppression:** To address this challenge, combination therapies that target the immunosuppressive components of the TME are being investigated. For example, combining mRNA vaccines with checkpoint inhibitors or other immunomodulatory agents may help overcome the immune-suppressive effects of the TME and enhance the efficacy of mRNA vaccines.

iii. **Manufacturing and Scalability:** One of the practical challenges facing mRNA cancer vaccines is the scalability of manufacturing.

Personalized mRNA vaccines, in particular, require the identification of unique neoantigens for each patient, which involves complex bioinformatics analysis and rapid production of customized mRNA sequences. While advances in mRNA manufacturing technology have made this process more feasible, large-scale production of personalized vaccines remains a logistical challenge.

- **Cost and Accessibility**: The cost of producing personalized mRNA vaccines is another limiting factor. As mRNA vaccines move toward broader clinical use, reducing the cost of production and ensuring accessibility to patients will be critical for their widespread adoption.

mRNA cancer vaccines represent a groundbreaking approach to cancer immunotherapy, offering the potential for highly personalized, safe, and effective treatments. Clinical trials have demonstrated the safety and immunogenicity of mRNA vaccines in several cancers, including melanoma, prostate cancer, and NSCLC (Liu et al., 2023). Success stories from early-phase trials and case studies highlight the ability of mRNA vaccines to induce durable anti-tumor responses and long-term immune memory. However, challenges such as tumor heterogeneity, delivery efficiency, and the immunosuppressive tumor microenvironment must be addressed to improve clinical outcomes. As ongoing trials continue to optimize mRNA vaccine design and combination therapies, the future of mRNA cancer vaccines holds great promise in revolutionizing cancer treatment.

7. Advantages and challenges

mRNA-based vaccines represent a transformative shift in the field of cancer immunotherapy, offering numerous advantages over conventional therapeutic approaches. By leveraging the body's natural protein synthesis mechanisms, mRNA vaccines can generate highly targeted immune responses against cancer-specific antigens, enabling precision medicine tailored to individual patients. However, despite these advantages, there are several challenges to the widespread implementation of mRNA vaccines, particularly in terms of stability, delivery, and overcoming immune evasion mechanisms employed by tumor cells. This article will explore the key advantages of mRNA-based cancer vaccines and delve into the challenges that must be addressed to realize their full potential in clinical settings.

7.1 Advantages over conventional therapies

i. **Rapid Development and Flexibility:** One of the most significant advantages of mRNA vaccines is their rapid development timeline. Traditional vaccine platforms, such as protein subunit or inactivated virus vaccines, typically require extensive time to produce, purify, and formulate antigenic components. In contrast, mRNA vaccines are based on synthetic production, which allows for much faster development (Acosta-Coley et al., 2022). The entire process of designing and producing an mRNA vaccine can be completed in weeks, rather than months or years, as seen with traditional vaccine approaches.

- **Adaptability to Emerging Antigens:** The modular nature of mRNA vaccine technology also provides unprecedented flexibility. The mRNA sequence encoding the target antigen can be easily modified or adjusted to reflect new or emerging antigens, making it a versatile platform for rapidly adapting to changes in the cancer's mutational landscape. This adaptability is crucial in oncology, where tumors can evolve and develop resistance to existing therapies. The ability to rapidly develop vaccines against newly discovered cancer antigens makes mRNA vaccines a highly responsive tool in cancer treatment.

- **Personalization for Cancer Therapy:** Another important advantage of mRNA vaccines is the potential for personalization. Personalized cancer vaccines can be developed to target specific neoantigens—mutations unique to an individual's tumor (Conniot et al., 2014). By identifying these tumor-specific mutations through sequencing technologies, mRNA vaccines can be customized to provoke an immune response tailored to the patient's cancer, making it a highly precise treatment strategy.

ii. **Precision and Specificity:** mRNA vaccines offer remarkable precision in targeting cancer cells. Traditional therapies like chemotherapy and radiation often have significant off-target effects, causing damage to healthy tissues along with cancer cells (Conniot et al., 2014). Immunotherapies, such as mRNA vaccines, aim to generate a specific immune response against cancer-specific antigens, thereby minimizing collateral damage to healthy cells.

- **Targeting Tumor-Specific Antigens:** The design of mRNA vaccines involves encoding TAAs or neoantigens, which are unique to cancer cells. This enables the immune system, particularly cytotoxic T cells (CD8$^+$), to recognize and destroy cancer cells expressing these antigens while sparing normal cells that do not express the target antigens (Labanieh et al., 2018). This level of specificity contrasts with the systemic toxicity often seen in conventional cancer treatments.

- **Potential for Combination Therapies:** mRNA vaccines also provide opportunities to be used in combination with other therapies, including checkpoint inhibitors and monoclonal antibodies, to enhance the overall efficacy of cancer treatment (Barbier et al., 2022). This precision medicine approach can synergize with other immune-modulating therapies to produce a robust, sustained immune response against cancer cells.

iii. **Immunogenicity and Safety Profile:** Another critical advantage of mRNA vaccines is their favorable safety profile and high immunogenicity, making them well-suited for cancer immunotherapy. Unlike DNA-based vaccines or viral vector-based vaccines, mRNA vaccines do not integrate into the host genome, thereby eliminating the risk of insertional mutagenesis or unintended genetic alterations.

- **High Immunogenicity:** mRNA vaccines are inherently immunogenic, meaning they can efficiently stimulate both the innate and adaptive immune systems. Upon delivery, mRNA molecules are taken up by APCs, such as dendritic cells, which translate the mRNA into antigenic proteins (Park et al., 2021). These proteins are then processed and presented on MHC molecules, stimulating T cells to mount a targeted immune response. This robust immune activation is a hallmark of mRNA vaccines and is one of the reasons they have shown promise in cancer therapy.

- **Safety of Synthetic mRNA:** The synthetic nature of mRNA molecules also makes them safer compared to live-attenuated or inactivated vaccines, which carry risks of reversion to a virulent form. mRNA vaccines are non-infectious and non-replicating, significantly reducing the risk of adverse effects. Moreover, the transient nature of mRNA ensures that once the encoded protein is expressed and the immune response is triggered, the mRNA is rapidly degraded by cellular mechanisms, further enhancing the safety profile.

iv. **Scalability and Manufacturing:** The simplicity of mRNA vaccine production is another key advantage, particularly for large-scale manufacturing. The production of mRNA involves chemical synthesis, which is faster and easier to scale compared to the biological production processes required for protein- or virus-based vaccines (Pascolo, 2004).

This scalability is crucial in ensuring that personalized cancer vaccines can be produced quickly and at a relatively low cost, making the technology accessible to a broader patient population.

- **Cost-Effective Production:** Because mRNA vaccines do not require live cells or complex fermentation processes, their manufacturing is less resource-intensive than traditional vaccines. Furthermore, the ability to produce large quantities of mRNA in a short time frame makes this platform ideal for rapidly meeting high demand, especially in the context of pandemic preparedness or large-scale cancer vaccine deployment.

7.2 Challenges: stability, delivery, and immune evasion

Despite these advantages, the development and clinical application of mRNA cancer vaccines face several significant challenges. Key obstacles include the intrinsic instability of mRNA, the need for effective delivery systems, and the ability of cancer cells to evade immune detection.

i. **Stability of mRNA Molecules:** One of the primary challenges in mRNA vaccine development is the inherent instability of mRNA molecules. mRNA is highly susceptible to degradation by ribonucleases (RNases), enzymes that are ubiquitous in the environment and within the human body (Blenke et al., 2023). The rapid degradation of mRNA can significantly reduce the efficacy of the vaccine, as the encoded antigen may not be produced in sufficient quantities to elicit a strong immune response.

- **Strategies to Improve Stability:** To overcome this challenge, researchers have employed several strategies to improve mRNA stability. One approach involves chemical modifications to the mRNA backbone, such as incorporating modified nucleosides (e.g., pseudouridine) that resist degradation by RNases. Additionally, mRNA can be encapsulated in LNPs, which protect the mRNA from enzymatic degradation while facilitating its delivery into cells (Blenke et al., 2023). These strategies have been critical in enhancing the stability and potency of mRNA vaccines, but further optimization is required to ensure long-term stability and efficacy.

ii. **Delivery Challenges:** Efficient delivery of mRNA into target cells, particularly APCs, is another major hurdle in mRNA vaccine development. Unlike small molecules or proteins, mRNA is a large, negatively charged molecule that cannot easily cross the cell membrane. As a result, effective delivery systems are needed to ensure that the mRNA reaches its target cells and is translated into the desired antigenic proteins.

- **Lipid Nanoparticles (LNPs):** The most widely used delivery system for mRNA vaccines is LNPs. LNPs are composed of lipids that form a protective shell around the mRNA, facilitating its uptake by cells through endocytosis (Eygeris et al., 2021). Once inside the cell, the LNPs release the mRNA, allowing it to be translated into antigenic proteins. LNPs have been highly successful in preclinical and clinical studies, but they are not without limitations. For instance, LNPs can induce inflammatory responses or trigger immune activation, which may lead to side effects (Żak and Zangi, 2021). Additionally, the efficiency of LNP-mediated delivery can vary depending on the tissue or cell type being targeted, and further refinement of LNP formulations is needed to optimize delivery.

- **Dendritic Cell Vaccines:** Another delivery strategy involves using DCs as carriers for mRNA vaccines. In this approach, patient-derived dendritic cells are transfected with mRNA encoding tumor antigens ex vivo and then re-infused into the patient. The dendritic cells present the tumor antigens to T cells, initiating a robust immune response (Perez and De Palma, 2019). While dendritic cell vaccines have shown promise in clinical trials, this approach is labor-intensive and costly, limiting its scalability. Moreover, the efficacy of dendritic cell vaccines can vary depending on the patient's immune status and the quality of the dendritic cells.

iii. **Immune Evasion by Tumor Cells:** One of the major challenges in cancer immunotherapy, including mRNA vaccines, is the ability of tumor cells to evade immune detection. Tumors employ several immune evasion strategies to suppress the immune response and avoid being targeted by the immune system (Umansky and Sevko, 2013).

- **Immunosuppressive Tumor Microenvironment:** Many tumors create an immunosuppressive microenvironment that inhibits the activity of T cells and other immune cells. Regulatory T cells (Tregs), myeloid-derived suppressor cells (MDSCs), and other immunosuppressive factors can prevent the immune system from effectively attacking the tumor, even if an mRNA vaccine successfully generates a strong immune response (Umansky and Sevko, 2013). To counteract this, mRNA vaccines are often combined with checkpoint inhibitors (e.g., anti-PD-1, anti-CTLA-4), which block the immunosuppressive signals and allow T cells to attack the tumor. While this combination has shown promise, overcoming the immunosuppressive tumor microenvironment remains a significant challenge in cancer immunotherapy.

- **Antigenic Escape:** Tumor cells can also evade immune detection through antigenic escape, a process in which they downregulate or mutate the target antigens recognized by T cells. This allows the tumor to avoid being destroyed by the immune system, even after vaccination (Jhunjhunwala et al., 2021). One potential solution is to design mRNA vaccines that target multiple antigens simultaneously, reducing the likelihood of antigenic escape. However, identifying the right combination of antigens remains a complex and ongoing area of research.

mRNA-based cancer vaccines offer numerous advantages over conventional therapies, including rapid development, precision targeting, and a favorable safety profile. Their ability to induce strong, specific immune responses makes them a promising tool in cancer immunotherapy. However, significant challenges remain, including the stability of mRNA molecules, the efficiency of delivery systems, and the ability to overcome immune evasion by tumor cells. Addressing these challenges will be critical to unlocking the full potential of mRNA vaccines in the fight against cancer.

8. Future directions and emerging innovations

mRNA cancer vaccines have opened a new frontier in immunotherapy, offering targeted, rapid, and flexible solutions for treating cancers such as melanoma. As this technology continues to evolve, several future directions and innovations are emerging that could further enhance the efficacy and applicability of mRNA vaccines. These next-generation approaches include combination therapies, personalized vaccines, expanding the use of mRNA vaccines to other cancer types beyond melanoma, and leveraging artificial intelligence (AI) and genomic profiling to optimize vaccine development.

a. **Next-Generation mRNA Vaccines:** The future of mRNA vaccines lies in advancing beyond the current generation of treatments, with a focus on enhancing their efficacy, broadening their scope, and improving patient outcomes. The most promising innovations include combination therapies and personalized cancer vaccines.

i. **Combination Therapies:** Combining mRNA vaccines with other therapeutic approaches is a key strategy to boost their effectiveness (Liu et al., 2018). This is particularly relevant in cancer, where the complexity of tumor biology often requires multi-pronged interventions to overcome immune evasion mechanisms.

- **Checkpoint Inhibitors:** Immune checkpoint inhibitors, such as anti-PD-1 and anti-CTLA-4, are being used in combination with mRNA vaccines to enhance immune responses. While mRNA vaccines can activate cytotoxic T cells ($CD8^+$), tumors often evade these immune responses by expressing checkpoint molecules that suppress T-cell activity (Haanen and Robert, 2015). By combining mRNA vaccines with checkpoint inhibitors, the immune system's ability to attack tumor cells is amplified. This synergy can result in more sustained and potent anti-tumor immunity.

- **Adjuvants and Cytokine Therapies:** Another combination strategy involves using immune-stimulating adjuvants or cytokines alongside mRNA vaccines. Adjuvants such as TLR agonists can be incorporated into the vaccine to enhance the activation of APCs and boost the overall immune response. Cytokines like interleukin-2 (IL-2) and interferon-alpha (IFN-α) can further enhance T-cell activation and proliferation, promoting a more robust immune attack on the tumor (Liu et al., 2018).

- **Oncolytic Viruses:** Oncolytic viruses, which selectively infect and kill cancer cells while stimulating an immune response, are another potential partner for mRNA vaccines. By combining these therapies, the viral infection can serve as a platform to release tumor antigens while simultaneously delivering mRNA vaccines that target specific cancer antigens. This could enhance the overall immunogenicity and lead to more effective tumor clearance.

ii. **Personalized mRNA Vaccines:** Personalization is a major emerging innovation in cancer treatment, and mRNA vaccines are particularly well-suited for this approach (Liu et al., 2018). Tumors often harbor unique mutations known as neoantigens, which can be targeted by the immune system. By tailoring mRNA vaccines to these neoantigens, personalized vaccines can be designed for each patient, leading to a highly specific immune response that targets the unique characteristics of the individual's cancer.

- **Neoantigen Identification:** Advances in genomic sequencing technologies have made it possible to identify patient-specific neoantigens. Once these neoantigens are discovered, mRNA vaccines can be designed to encode these precise antigens, priming the immune system to recognize and destroy tumor cells expressing them. Personalized mRNA vaccines are already being tested in clinical trials, and early results suggest that they can elicit strong anti-tumor immune responses with minimal off-target effects.
- **Rapid Vaccine Design:** The modular nature of mRNA vaccines allows for the rapid design and production of personalized vaccines. With the advent of automated synthesis platforms, mRNA vaccines can be developed and produced in a matter of weeks, making personalized cancer treatment more accessible and feasible in clinical settings. As sequencing and vaccine synthesis technologies continue to improve, the time between cancer diagnosis and the delivery of a personalized vaccine is expected to shorten further.

b. **Potential for Other Cancers Beyond Melanoma:** While much of the current focus has been on melanoma, mRNA vaccines have the potential to treat a broad range of cancers. Their versatility and ability to target multiple antigens make them applicable to various tumor types, particularly those with high mutational burdens or known cancer-specific antigens.

   i. **Lung Cancer:** Non-small cell lung cancer (NSCLC) is one of the most common and lethal cancers, and the development of mRNA vaccines for this disease is an area of active research. NSCLC often expresses specific oncogenic mutations, such as EGFR or KRAS mutations, which can be targeted by mRNA vaccines (Uras et al., 2020). Early preclinical studies have shown promise, and clinical trials are underway to assess the efficacy of mRNA vaccines in lung cancer patients.

   ii. **Prostate and Breast Cancers:** Prostate and breast cancers, which are often driven by hormone-related mechanisms, have also become potential targets for mRNA vaccines. In prostate cancer, for example, mRNA vaccines could target the prostate-specific antigen (PSA), a protein highly expressed in prostate cancer cells (Dannull et al., 2000). Similarly, in breast cancer, mRNA vaccines could be designed to target HER2 or other oncogenes associated with tumor progression. Combination therapies with hormone blockers or immune checkpoint inhibitors may further enhance the efficacy of mRNA vaccines in these cancers.

iii. **Hematologic Malignancies:** Hematologic cancers, such as leukemia and lymphoma, also present an opportunity for mRNA vaccine development. These cancers are characterized by the overexpression of specific antigens, such as BCR-ABL in chronic myeloid leukemia or CD19 in B-cell lymphomas (Braun and Wu, 2017). By designing mRNA vaccines to target these antigens, it is possible to elicit a strong immune response against cancerous cells. The advantage in hematologic malignancies lies in the accessibility of cancer cells to the immune system, potentially enhancing the effectiveness of mRNA vaccines.

c. **Integration with AI and Genomic Profiling for Vaccine Development:** The future of mRNA vaccine development will likely involve advanced computational tools and data-driven approaches (McCaffrey, 2022). By integrating artificial intelligence (AI) and genomic profiling technologies, researchers can accelerate the design and optimization of mRNA vaccines, improving their efficacy and personalization.

i. **AI-Driven Vaccine Design:** AI has the potential to revolutionize mRNA vaccine design by optimizing the selection of target antigens and improving the overall structure of mRNA constructs (McCaffrey, 2022). Machine learning algorithms can analyze vast datasets of tumor genomic information to identify the most immunogenic and tumor-specific neoantigens. These algorithms can predict which antigens are most likely to elicit a strong immune response, enabling researchers to prioritize the best candidates for mRNA vaccine development.

- **Predictive Models for Immune Response:** AI can also be used to build predictive models that simulate the immune system's response to different antigens. By incorporating data on T-cell receptor recognition, antigen processing, and presentation, AI tools can provide insights into how the immune system will respond to an mRNA vaccine before it even reaches clinical trials. This can save time and resources by eliminating candidates that are unlikely to succeed in later stages of development.

ii. **Genomic Profiling for Personalized Vaccines:** The integration of genomic profiling with mRNA vaccine technology represents a powerful approach for developing personalized cancer treatments. By sequencing a patient's tumor, researchers can identify unique mutations and neoantigens that serve as the basis for a personalized mRNA vaccine (Sahin and Türeci, 2018).

- **Next-Generation Sequencing (NGS):** The use of NGS allows for comprehensive profiling of a tumor's mutational landscape, identifying not only driver mutations but also passenger mutations that may serve as neoantigens. By combining NGS with AI-driven analysis, researchers can quickly identify the most relevant antigens for vaccine development (Kiyotani et al., 2021).
- **Multi-Omics Integration:** Beyond just genomic data, integrating other "omics" data—such as transcriptomics, proteomics, and metabolomics—into the vaccine development process could further enhance personalization. By analyzing a tumor's gene expression patterns and protein levels, researchers can gain a more holistic understanding of the tumor microenvironment and design vaccines that are optimized for each patient's unique cancer profile (Chakraborty et al., 2024).

The future of mRNA cancer vaccines is incredibly promising, with ongoing innovations aimed at improving their efficacy, personalization, and applicability to various cancers. Next-generation vaccines, particularly those involving combination therapies and personalized approaches, are poised to significantly enhance the outcomes of cancer immunotherapy. Furthermore, expanding the use of mRNA vaccines beyond melanoma to other cancer types could revolutionize the treatment landscape for multiple malignancies. Finally, the integration of AI and genomic profiling holds immense potential for optimizing vaccine development, enabling faster, more effective, and personalized cancer treatments. As these technologies continue to evolve, mRNA cancer vaccines are expected to play an increasingly prominent role in the future of oncology.

9. Conclusion

mRNA vaccines represent a groundbreaking advancement in the treatment of melanoma and other cancers, offering a versatile, rapid, and highly targeted approach to cancer immunotherapy. Recent progress has significantly improved our understanding of the mechanisms by which mRNA vaccines function, leading to effective treatments for various cancers, with melanoma being the primary focus. These vaccines stimulate potent immune responses by encoding tumor-specific antigens and offer the flexibility to adapt constructs quickly, positioning them at the forefront of cancer treatment innovations. The potential of mRNA vaccines in melanoma treatment is substantial, targeting tumor antigens with precision, activating both innate and adaptive immune responses, and breaking immune tolerance that tumors often exploit. Melanoma, a highly immunogenic cancer, serves as an ideal platform for developing mRNA vaccines due to its high mutational burden, generating numerous neoantigens that can be targeted by the immune system. These vaccines encode antigens that directly induce antigen-specific $CD4^+$ and $CD8^+$ T cell responses, which are essential for attacking and eradicating melanoma cells.

A key advantage of mRNA vaccines in melanoma treatment is their rapid development and customization. Because these vaccines are synthetic and do not rely on live viruses or cell cultures, they can be produced quickly and modified to target specific mutations or antigens. This adaptability is especially useful in melanoma, where each patient's tumor may have unique genetic mutations driving cancer progression. Personalized mRNA vaccines, tailored to an individual's tumor profile, are emerging as a promising strategy for eliciting highly specific immune responses. Additionally, mRNA vaccines offer several advantages over traditional cancer therapies. Unlike conventional treatments such as chemotherapy or radiation, which can have non-specific effects and cause significant damage to healthy tissues, mRNA vaccines are designed to target only cancer cells. This specificity reduces the risk of severe side effects and improves the overall safety profile. Furthermore, mRNA vaccines can be used in combination with other immunotherapies, such as immune checkpoint inhibitors, enhancing the immune system's ability to recognize and eliminate melanoma cells. As the field of mRNA vaccines evolves, several future directions hold promise for enhancing their efficacy and expanding their use beyond melanoma. One of the most exciting areas of development is the ongoing refinement of personalized cancer vaccines. By leveraging advancements in genomic sequencing and neoantigen identification, researchers are increasingly able to design vaccines customized to target the specific mutations in a patient's tumor. This personalized approach has the potential to revolutionize cancer treatment, offering highly specific therapies tailored to the genetic makeup of each patient's cancer.

Another promising avenue for future development is integrating mRNA vaccines with combination therapies. The success of combining mRNA vaccines with immune checkpoint inhibitors in clinical trials highlights the potential for multi-modal approaches. Combining mRNA vaccines with therapies that modulate the tumor microenvironment, such as oncolytic viruses or cytokine therapies that enhance immune activation, could lead to more robust and sustained anti-tumor responses. These combination strategies offer a means of overcoming immune evasion and resistance, common challenges in cancer treatment. Expanding the use of mRNA vaccines to other types of cancers is another critical area of research. While melanoma has been the focus of mRNA vaccine development due to its immunogenicity, the versatility of mRNA technology makes it applicable to a wide range of cancers. Tumors with high mutational burdens, such as lung, colorectal, and bladder cancers, as well as cancers with specific known antigens, such as prostate and breast cancers, are prime candidates for mRNA vaccine development. As research progresses, it is likely that mRNA vaccines will become a cornerstone of immunotherapy across various cancer types. Advances in delivery technologies and stability will play a crucial role in the future success of mRNA vaccines. LNP formulations have shown great promise in effectively delivering mRNA vaccines to target tissues. However, ongoing research aims to further optimize these delivery platforms to improve stability, reduce degradation, and enhance immune responses. Innovations in delivery systems, such as incorporating adjuvants or designing more stable mRNA constructs, will be key to improving the efficacy and durability of mRNA vaccines in clinical settings. Looking ahead, the integration of advanced technologies such as artificial intelligence (AI) and machine learning into the vaccine development process is poised to accelerate advancements. AI can be used to optimize the selection of tumor antigens, predict immune responses, and design mRNA constructs that elicit the most effective immune activation. By analyzing large datasets of patient-specific genomic and immunological information, AI-driven tools can help refine and personalize cancer vaccine development, making treatments more precise and tailored to individual needs. In conclusion, mRNA vaccines demonstrate enormous potential in melanoma treatment and are poised to play a significant role in the future of cancer immunotherapy. Their ability to induce robust and specific immune responses, combined with rapid development and personalization capabilities, makes them a powerful tool in the fight against cancer. As the field continues to evolve, innovations in personalized vaccines, combination therapies, and delivery platforms, along with AI integration and genomic profiling, will drive the development of next-generation mRNA vaccines. These advancements hold the promise of transforming not only melanoma treatment but also the broader landscape of cancer immunotherapy, offering new hope for patients across various cancer types.

References

Acosta-Coley, I., et al. (2022). Vaccines platforms and COVID-19: What you need to know. *Tropical Diseases, Travel Medicine and Vaccines, 8*(1), 20.

American Cancer Society Cancer Facts & Statistics. http://cancerstatisticscenter.cancer.org/ (accessed 13th October 2024.

Bahar, M. E., Kim, H. J., & Kim, D. R. (2023). Targeting the RAS/RAF/MAPK pathway for cancer therapy: From mechanism to clinical studies. *Signal Transduction and Targeted Therapy, 8*(1), 455. https://doi.org/10.1038/s41392-023-01705-z.

Barbier, A. J., Jiang, A. Y., Zhang, P., Wooster, R., & Anderson, D. G. (2022). The clinical progress of mRNA vaccines and immunotherapies. *Nature Biotechnology, 40*(6), 840–854.

Beck, J. D., et al. (2021). mRNA therapeutics in cancer immunotherapy. *Molecular Cancer, 20*(1), 69.

Bidram, M., et al. (2021). mRNA-based cancer vaccines: A therapeutic strategy for the treatment of melanoma patients. *Vaccines (Basel), 9*(10), https://doi.org/10.3390/vaccines9101060.

Blenke, E. O., et al. (2023). The storage and in-use stability of mRNA vaccines and therapeutics: Not a cold case. *Journal of Pharmaceutical Sciences, 112*(2), 386–403.

Braun, D. A., & Wu, C. J. (2017). Antigen discovery and therapeutic targeting in hematologic malignancies. *The Cancer Journal, 23*(2), 115–124.

Cafri, G., et al. (2020). mRNA vaccine–induced neoantigen-specific T cell immunity in patients with gastrointestinal cancer. *Journal of Clinical Investigation, 130*(11), 5976–5988. https://doi.org/10.1172/JCI134915.

Carreno, B. M., et al. (2015). A dendritic cell vaccine increases the breadth and diversity of melanoma neoantigen-specific T cells. *Science (New York, N. Y.), 348*(6236), 803–808. https://doi.org/10.1126/science.aaa3828.

Chakraborty, S., Sharma, G., Karmakar, S., & Banerjee, S. (2024). Multi-OMICS approaches in cancer biology: New era in cancer therapy. *Biochimica et Biophysica Acta (BBA)-Molecular Basis of Disease, 1870*(5), 167120.

Conniot, J., et al. (2014). Cancer immunotherapy: Nanodelivery approaches for immune cell targeting and tracking. *Frontiers in Chemistry, 2*, 105.

Cui, J.-W., et al. (2024). Tumor immunotherapy resistance: Revealing the mechanism of PD-1/PD-L1-mediated tumor immune escape. *Biomedicine & Pharmacotherapy, 171*, 116203. https://doi.org/10.1016/j.biopha.2024.116203.

Dannull, J., et al. (2000). Prostate stem cell antigen is a promising candidate for immunotherapy of advanced prostate cancer. *Cancer Research, 60*(19), 5522–5528.

Deng, Z., Tian, Y., Song, J., An, G., & Yang, P. (2022). mRNA vaccines: The dawn of a new era of cancer immunotherapy (in English). *Frontiers in Immunology, Review, 13*. https://doi.org/10.3389/fimmu.2022.887125.

Eygeris, Y., Gupta, M., Kim, J., & Sahay, G. (2021). Chemistry of lipid nanoparticles for RNA delivery. *Accounts of Chemical Research, 55*(1), 2–12.

Haanen, J. B., & Robert, C. (2015). Immune checkpoint inhibitors. *Immuno-Oncology, 42*, 55–66.

He, M., et al. (2023). Unleashing novel horizons in advanced prostate cancer treatment: investigating the potential of prostate specific membrane antigen-targeted nanomedicine-based combination therapy. *Frontiers in Immunology, 14*, 1265751.

Jhunjhunwala, S., Hammer, C., & Delamarre, L. (2021). Antigen presentation in cancer: Insights into tumour immunogenicity and immune evasion. *Nature Reviews. Cancer, 21*(5), 298–312.

Kiyotani, K., Toyoshima, Y., & Nakamura, Y. (2021). Immunogenomics in personalized cancer treatments. *Journal of Human Genetics, 66*(9), 901–907.

Labanieh, L., Majzner, R. G., & Mackall, C. L. (2018). Programming CAR-T cells to kill cancer. *Nature Biomedical Engineering, 2*(6), 377–391.

Lao, Y., Shen, D., Zhang, W., He, R., & Jiang, M. (2022). Immune checkpoint inhibitors in cancer therapy—How to overcome drug resistance? *Cancers, 14*(15), 3575.

Le, D. T., Pardoll, D. M., & Jaffee, E. M. (2010). Cellular vaccine approaches. *Cancer Journal, Review, 16*(4), 304–310. https://doi.org/10.1097/PPO.0b013e3181eb33d7.

Liu, L., et al. (2018). Combination immunotherapy of MUC1 mRNA nano-vaccine and CTLA-4 blockade effectively inhibits growth of triple negative breast cancer. *Molecular Therapy, 26*(1), 45–55.

Liu, C., Shi, Q., Huang, X., Koo, S., Kong, N., & Tao, W. (2023). mRNA-based cancer therapeutics. *Nature Reviews. Cancer, 23*(8), 526–543.

Li, X., Ma, S., Gao, T., Mai, Y., Song, Z., & Yang, J. (2022). The main battlefield of mRNA vaccine–Tumor immune microenvironment. *International Immunopharmacology, 113*, 109367.

Li, J., Zhang, Y., Yang, Y.-G., & Sun, T. (2024). Advancing mRNA therapeutics: the role and future of nanoparticle delivery systems. *Molecular Pharmaceutics, 21*(8), 3743–3763.

McCaffrey, P. (2022). Artificial intelligence for vaccine design. *Vaccine Design: Methods and Protocols, Volume 3. Resources for Vaccine Development,* 3–13.

Miao, L., Zhang, Y., & Huang, L. (2021). mRNA vaccine for cancer immunotherapy. *Molecular Cancer, 20*(1), 41.

Mohanty, R., Chowdhury, C. R., Arega, S., Sen, P., Ganguly, P., & Ganguly, N. (2019). CAR T cell therapy: A new era for cancer treatment. *Oncology Reports, 42*(6), 2183–2195.

Park, J. W., Lagniton, P. N., Liu, Y., & Xu, R.-H. (2021). mRNA vaccines for COVID-19: What, why and how. *International Journal of Biological Sciences, 17*(6), 1446.

Pascolo, S. (2004). Messenger RNA-based vaccines. *Expert Opinion on Biological Therapy, 4*(8), 1285–1294.

Perez, C. R., & De Palma, M. (2019). Engineering dendritic cell vaccines to improve cancer immunotherapy. *Nature Communications, 10*(1), 5408.

Rojas, L. A., et al. (2023). Personalized RNA neoantigen vaccines stimulate T cells in pancreatic cancer. *Nature, 618*(7963), 144–150. https://doi.org/10.1038/s41586-023-06063-y.

Sahin, U., & Türeci, Ö. (2018). Personalized vaccines for cancer immunotherapy. *Science (New York, N. Y.), 359*(6382), 1355–1360.

Sayour, E. J., Boczkowski, D., Mitchell, D. A., & Nair, S. K. (2024). Cancer mRNA vaccines: Clinical advances and future opportunities. *Nature Reviews Clinical Oncology,* 1–12.

Shirley, C. A., Chhabra, G., Amiri, D., Chang, H., & Ahmad, N. (2024). Immune escape and metastasis mechanisms in melanoma: Breaking down the dichotomy (in English). *Frontiers in Immunology, Review, 15*. https://doi.org/10.3389/fimmu.2024.1336023.

Song, Q., Zhang, C.-D., & Wu, X.-H. (2018). Therapeutic cancer vaccines: From initial findings to prospects. *Immunology Letters, 196*, 11–21. https://doi.org/10.1016/j.imlet.2018.01.011.

Umansky, V., & Sevko, A. (2013). Tumor microenvironment and myeloid-derived suppressor cells. *Cancer Microenvironment, 6*, 169–177.

Uras, I. Z., Moll, H. P., & Casanova, E. (2020). Targeting KRAS mutant non-small-cell lung cancer: Past, present and future. *International Journal of Molecular Sciences, 21*(12), 4325.

Wang, B., Pei, J., Xu, S., Liu, J., & Yu, J. (2023). Recent advances in mRNA cancer vaccines: Meeting challenges and embracing opportunities (in English). *Frontiers in Immunology, Review, 14*. https://doi.org/10.3389/fimmu.2023.1246682.

Wei, J., & Hui, A.-M. (2022). The paradigm shift in treatment from Covid-19 to oncology with mRNA vaccines. *Cancer Treatment Reviews, 107*. https://doi.org/10.1016/j.ctrv.2022.102405.

Xie, N., Shen, G., Gao, W., Huang, Z., Huang, C., & Fu, L. (2023). Neoantigens: Promising targets for cancer therapy. *Signal transduction and targeted therapy, 8*(1), 9.

Zhang, Z., et al. (2021). Neoantigen: A new breakthrough in tumor immunotherapy. *Frontiers in Immunology, 12*, 672356.

Żak, M. M., & Zangi, L. (2021). Lipid nanoparticles for organ-specific mRNA therapeutic delivery. *Pharmaceutics, 13*(10), 1675.

CHAPTER SIX

Therapeutic mRNAs for cancer immunotherapy: From structure to delivery

Monika Vishwakarma[a,b], Wasim Akram[c,*], and Tanweer Haider[d,*]

[a]Department of Pharmaceutical Sciences, Doctor Harisingh Gour University, Sagar, Madhya Pradesh, India
[b]Faculty of Pharmacy, Kalinga University, Naya Raipur, Chhattisgarh, India
[c]Amity Institute of Pharmacy, Amity University Madhya Pradesh, Gwalior, Madhya Pradesh, India
[d]Gyan Vihar School of Pharmacy, Suresh Gyan Vihar University, Jaipur, Rajasthan, India
*Corresponding authors. e-mail address: wasimjiwaji@gmail.com; tanweer0852@gmail.com

Contents

Abstract

mRNA carries genetic information and is used for the synthesis of proteins, fragments of proteins, and peptides in the scope of biotechnology and medicine. Once introduced into cells, this mRNA gets translated into a corresponding protein with cellular machinery. All kinds of mRNA encoding any protein, peptide, and fragment of proteins have been designed to be used for various therapeutic goals, including cancerous diseases, immunotherapy, vaccine preparation, tissue engineering, and genetic disorders, among others. These vaccines encode tumor-specific antigens that stimulate the immune system to recognize and attack cancer cells. Additionally, mRNA can be designed to produce proteins that modulate immune checkpoints, thereby enhancing the immune system's ability to target cancer cells. Synthetic mRNA can also engineer immune cells, such as T cells, to improve their cancer-fighting capabilities. For instance, mRNA can be engineered to generate CAR T cells targeting specific antigens that are expressed in the cancer. Designed mRNA can encode functional proteins in patients suffering from genetic disorders characterized by an

Advances in Immunology, Volume 165
ISSN 0065-2776, https://doi.org/10.1016/bs.ai.2024.10.013

absence or defect in a particular protein. However, mRNA is intrinsically unstable and may require special mechanisms to protect it from degradation. mRNA delivery to target cells remains a challenge. Engineered nanocarriers containing mRNA can improve the efficiency and enable the delivery to specific sites, that can provide a stimulant or substance for therapeutic purposes. This combination may improve their stability and efficacy in multiple applications of therapies. The following chapter throws light on basic advances in mRNA-based cancer therapy and provides insights into the nanotherapeutics using mRNA in key preclinical developments and the evolving clinical landscape.

1. Introduction

According to the World Health Organization, cancer is one of the most serious health problems of by the International Agency for Research on Cancer, cancer incidence is expected to increase exponentially (77 %, no less), and more than 35 million new cases will be registered in 2050, up from the estimated 20 million cases in 2022 (Who, 2024). Chemotherapy, surgical procedures and radiotherapy cancer treatments are readily available. However, the efficiency and effectiveness of conventional cancer treatments are limited by several challenges, including drug resistance, poor drug penetration, limited ability to reach the tumor microenvironment, lack of tumor specificity, and toxicity to normal cells. These issues hinder the ability of these treatments to eradicate cancer cells, reducing their overall therapeutic potential (Haider, Tiwari, Vyas, & Soni, 2019; Haider, Pandey, Banjare, Gupta, & Soni, 2020). To enhance the effectiveness of treatments, improve accuracy, and avoid harming healthier cells, researchers are always on the lookout for new methods and innovations in cancer therapy. Recent advancements in cancer treatment encompass breakthroughs like stem cell therapy (Chu et al., 2020), targeted therapies (Haider & Soni, 2022, Haider, Pandey et al., 2020; Pandey, Haider, Chandak et al., 2020), ablation techniques (De Baere & Deschamps, 2014; Debela et al., 2021), nanoparticle-based treatments (Adnan et al., 2023, Haider et al., 2022, Singhai et al., 2023; Vishwakarma, Haider, & Soni, 2024), natural antioxidants (Chahal, Saini, Chhillar, & Saini, 2018), prodrugs nanomedicine (Pandey, Haider, Gour, Soni, & Gupta, 2020; Yang, Gao, Pei, Xu, & Yu, 2020), radionics (Andreadis et al., 2004), chemodynamic therapy (Wang, Zhong, Liu, & Cheng, 2020), sonodynamic therapy (Mchale, Callan, Nomikou, Fowley, & Callan, 2016), ferroptosis-based therapies (Luo et al., 2021), immunotherapy (Chang et al., 2024, Jana, He, Chen, Liu, & Zhao, 2024; You et al., 2024), etc.

Several cellular and molecular processes allow cancer cells to evade the host's immune response. These include downregulating MHC molecules on their surface, expressing immune checkpoint proteins such as PD-L1, secreting immunosuppressive factors, altering the machinery for antigen presentation, and creating a tumor microenvironment that inhibits T cell activation (Gupta et al., 2023). Cancer immunotherapy relies on the body's natural immunity, which has shown great potential. There are several strategies to improve the immune system in cancer such as cytokine therapy (Propper & Balkwill, 2022)Monoclonal antibody (MAb) therapy (Delgado & Garcia-Sanz, 2023), checkpoint inhibitors (Bagchi, Yuan, & Engleman, 2021), adaptive T cell engineering, and therapies (Ellis, Sheppard, & Riley, 2021), cancer vaccines (Saxena, Van Der Burg, Melief, & Bhardwaj, 2021) and combination immune therapy (Yap et al., 2021).

Messenger RNA (mRNA) vaccines and therapies are among the potential therapies in cancer immunotherapy. In recent years, we have witnessed a rise in the use of mRNA for therapeutic purposes, especially in vaccines and immunotherapy. The recent successes of mRNA vaccines in controlling COVID-19 have significantly accelerated these advancements (Hussain et al., 2022). This new era has now brought mRNA technology for various types of cancers. The advantage of mRNA-based therapies lies in the direct harnessing of the natural protein synthesis machinery to stimulate the immune system to recognize and eliminate tumor cells. Moreover, mRNA therapy can encode a broad spectrum of tumor-specific antigens, immune modulators, and chimeric antigen receptors (CARs) in a manner that promotes personalized and targeted approaches to cancer treatment (Sun, Zhang, Wang, Yang, & Xu, 2023).

mRNA is a single-stranded molecule that acts as a mediator between DNA and protein synthesis. mRNA carries genetic information from the DNA located in the cell's nucleus to the ribosome, where proteins are assembled (N. Kuhn et al., 2012). The idea of using mRNA as a therapeutic tool emerged several years ago; however, it faced enormous technical challenges, mainly due to the instability of mRNA and its rapid degradation by the body's nucleases. The highly unstable nature of mRNA and inefficient delivery methods have kept the application of such species in medicine at a very low level (Li. Liu et al., 2023). Over the past two decades, that antagonism has been well addressed by aggressive research and development, which has yielded messengers with high stability and efficiency. Advanced mRNA synthesis, processing, and delivery have introduced potential therapeutic benefits of mRNA. Current challenges that mRNA can address include infectious diseases, cancer, and genetic disorders (Qin et al., 2022). One of the major advantages of mRNA therapies is their ability to induce the synthesis of almost any protein in the body. Researchers design synthetic mRNA sequences, after which they can command cells to produce the antigen-specific protein of interest for an immune response against cancer cells. The main feature of mRNA vaccines is encoding tumor antigens for the immune system to attack cancer cells (Wang et al., 2021).

The success of mRNA-based vaccines in cancer immunotherapy depends on their ability to stimulate immune responses that specifically target tumor cells (Li, Wang, Peng et al., 2023). This process begins with the introduction into the body of synthetic mRNA encoding a tumor-specific antigen. Once inside cells, the mRNA is translated into corresponding proteins displayed on the cell surface by major histocompatibility complex (MHC) molecules. This tumor antigen presentation activates both innate and adaptive immune responses, leading to the recruitment of cytotoxic T cells, which recognize and eliminate cancer cells (Beck et al., 2021). In addition to encoding tumor antigens, mRNA-based therapies can be designed to produce proteins that regulate immune checkpoints, such as programmed death ligand 1 (PD-L1) and lymphocyte-associated protein 4 (CTLA-4) (Pandey, Young, Kumar, & Jain, 2022). By inhibiting these immune checkpoints, mRNA treatments can enhance the body's ability to mount an effective immune response against cancer cells. In addition, mRNA can be used to engineer immune cells, such as T cells, using chimeric antigen receptor (CAR) technology. CAR T cells are genetically modified to express receptors that specifically recognize and bind to antigens on the surface of tumor cells, leading to their destruction (Mavi et al., 2023).

mRNA-based therapeutic agents have a high potential to be the safest therapeutic drugs. In DNA-based therapies, the concern is the possibility of integration into the host genome as well as the possibility of mutation (Hosseinkhani, Domb, Sharifzadeh, & Nahum, 2023). On the other hand, mRNA is not incorporated into DNA. It is degraded by the cell itself after translation to produce proteins, thereby reducing the risk factor behind such therapeutic applications (Sahin, Karikó, & Türeci, 2014). Another major advantage of mRNA therapies is flexibility and versatility (Qin et al., 2022). The ease with which mRNA sequences encoding such a wide range of proteins can be designed and synthesized allows for highly personalized therapies (Al Fayez et al., 2023).

However, this therapy faces several challenges, particularly in effectively getting the mRNA into the cells. The challenge is that mRNA is unstable and can also be degraded by ribonucleases, so it will require a delivery system to protect itself from degradation and be effectively endocytosed by cells (Wadhwa, Aljabbari, Lokras, Foged, & Thakur, 2020). Targeted and nanosized drug delivery carriers are used to overcome these hurdles in mRNA therapy. Nanocarrier systems (NCs) are nanoparticles and nanovesicles designed to deliver drugs, genetic materials, peptides, and other substances directly to specific target sites for the treatment of various diseases (Haider, Pandey, Sandha, Gupta, & Soni, 2020). The size and structure of the NCs are important for effective mRNA delivery. In this regard, scientists have tested different ways to tune the size, charge, and surface characteristics of NCs to achieve improved biodistribution, cellular uptake, and immune responses. Lipid nanoparticles (LNPs) are one of the most efficient delivery systems identified so far for mRNA vaccines (Ramachandran, Satapathy, & Dutta, 2022). LNPs encapsulate the mRNA, protecting it from degradation and allowing it to reach the target cells. When the mRNA enters the cells, it is released from the nanoparticles and converted into the protein it matches (Hou, Zaks, Langer, & Dong, 2021). Other systems in development include polymeric nanoparticles (Neshat et al., 2023), solid-lipid nanoparticles (SLNs) (Choi et al., 2008), and hybrid nanoparticles (Gao et al., 2021), which aim to improve mRNA stability and therapy efficacy. These protect mRNA from degradation and can be delivered to specific tissues or targeted to particular immune cells, such as dendritic cells (Cifuentes-Rius, Desai, Yuen, Johnston, & Voelcker, 2021). In immunotherapy, dendritic cells are central to antigen presentation and T cell activation, and targeting them, along with their cognate T cells, is considered an important target in cancer therapy (Palucka & Banchereau, 2012).

This chapter delves into the foundational aspects of mRNA therapeutics, emphasizing their role in cancer immunotherapy. The chapter explores the structure and pharmacology of mRNA, its therapeutic applications, and the challenges and innovations in its delivery systems. Additionally, this chapter highlights the recent advancements in preclinical and clinical trials and the potential of mRNA technology to revolutionize cancer treatment.

1.1 Structure and pharmacology of mRNA

The main object of mRNA is the transfer of genetic information from the nucleus's DNA to the cytoplasmic ribosome for the translation process of protein synthesis. mRNA precursors are synthesized during transcription as a complementary strand to the template strand of DNA. Afterwards, the introns are spliced out of the precursor mRNA, a 5′ cap is added, the 3′ end is polyadenylated, and the mature mRNA is transported out of the nucleus. The mRNA molecule recruits ribosomes in the cytoplasm, and translation is initiated. (Labster Theory Pages, 2024). mRNA has many structure components which play crucial roles in its stability, cellular localization, and translation. The mRNA's structure has many key components such as 5′cap, 5′ untranslated region (5′ UTR), Open Reading Frame (ORF), also known as Coding Region, 3′ Untranslated Region (3′ UTR), and Poly (A) Tail (Fig. 1). Whereas some other applications of mRNA have also been identified by researchers for therapeutic application, understanding the mRNA's structure is essential for understanding its expression and pharmacological effects. Below is a brief description of the structure components of mRNA and its function.

1.1.1 5′cap

The 5′ cap is a guanosine nucleotide having a methyl group at the 7-position, sometimes written as m7G. The cap is linked through a triphosphate bond (PPP) to the initial nucleotide at the 5′ terminus of mRNA, where transcription commences (the +1 position). The 5′ mRNA cap enhances ribosome binding during translation and protects it from destruction. The primary 5′ cap structure in mRNA is a cap-0 structure. In eukaryotes, the first nucleotide (+1) next to the 5′ cap can undergo further

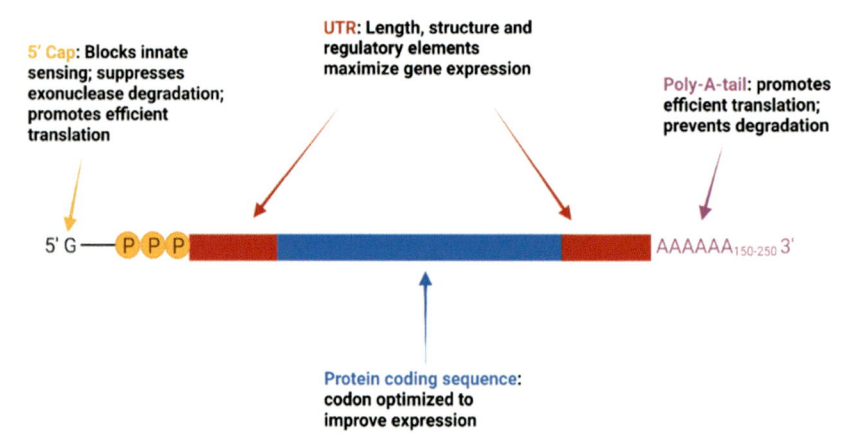

Fig. 1 The key components of mRNA structure. Figure republished by Cacicedo, Limeres, and Gehring (2022) through Creative Commons Attribution (CC BY) license.

modification to form a cap-1 structure, which diminishes immunogenicity. A 5′ cap-0 structure arises when the next nucleotide remains unmodified. Adding a methyl group to the first nucleotide forms a cap-1 structure. The cap-1 structure differentiates self from nonself, resulting in reduced immunogenicity when delivered in vivo (Takara, 2024).

1.1.2 5′ Untranslated region (5′ UTR)

The sequences on either side of a gene's coding sequence are known as untranslated regions or UTRs. They don't encode amino acids, yet they are transcribed to pre-mRNA nonetheless (Spurna et al., 2022). Upstream ORFs (uORFs), internal ribosome entry sites, microRNA binding sites, and structural features essential in the control of mRNA stability, pre-mRNA splicing, and translation initiation are all found in abundance in the 5′ untranslated region of mRNA domain (Hinnebusch, Ivanov, & Sonenberg, 2016).

1.1.3 Open reading frame

The term "open reading frame" refers to a frame of reference and the RNA code that the ribosomes are "reading" to produce a protein (Eisenhut et al., 2023). Furthermore, "open" indicates that the ribosome can continue reading the RNA code and add additional amino acids one after the other. Although a repetitive sequence of As, Cs, Ts, and Gs, DNA has a language of its own that is translated into RNA and subsequently into proteins. Additionally, the mRNA reads three letters simultaneously during translation into a protein rather than one letter at a time. And each of those three letters—whether the ribosome interprets a AAA, UUU, or AUG, the molecular apparatus that will form the protein as a specific amino acid. These three letters are known as codons. Thus, one amino acid is coded by AUG, another by UUU, and so on. Therefore, an open reading frame is the length of transcribed DNA or RNA that allows the ribosome to move through and add amino acids one at a time until it reaches a codon that is devoid of all amino acid coding. The ribosome pauses when it occurs because it becomes confused. A stop codon closes the frame for open reading (Shchelochkov, 2024).

1.1.4 3′ Untranslated region (3′ UTR)

The noncoding portions of mRNAs are known as 3′ untranslated regions (3′-UTRs). 3′-UTRs are best recognized for regulating mRNA fates like degradation, translation, and localization, but they can also operate as long noncoding or short RNAs, as evidenced by studies on both full 3′-UTRs and cleaved fragments (Mayr, 2017). Furthermore, 3′-UTRs regulate protein-protein interactions, allowing them to convey genetic information contained in 3′ UTRs to proteins. This function has been shown to influence various protein characteristics, such as protein complex formation and posttranslational modifications, but it is also expected to affect protein conformations. As a result, 3′ UTR-mediated information transfer can influence protein properties that are not encoded in the amino acid sequence (Mayr, 2019).

1.1.5 Poly (A) Tail

The poly-A tail is an extended sequence of adenine nucleotides appended to a messenger RNA (mRNA) molecule during RNA processing to enhance the molecule's stability (Passmore & Coller, 2022). Upon transcription of a gene in a eukaryotic cell, the resultant RNA molecule undergoes a series of alterations referred to as RNA processing (Licatalosi & Darnell, 2010). These changes modify both termini of the initial RNA transcript to generate a mature mRNA molecule. A poly-A tail is added at the 3′ end of the RNA molecule. The 3′ end of the transcript is cleaved to release a 3′ hydroxyl group. Subsequently, an enzyme known as poly-A polymerase appends a sequence of adenine nucleotides to the RNA. The process known as polyadenylation adds a poly-A tail consisting of 100 to 250 residues. The poly-A tail enhances the stability of the RNA molecule and inhibits its destruction. Furthermore, the poly-A tail facilitates the export of the mature messenger RNA molecule from the nucleus and its subsequent translation into a protein by ribosomes in the cytoplasm (Scitable, 2024).

1.2 Modification in mRNA

Despite identifying the initial chemical changes in mRNA over 40 years ago, its functional importance has only recently started to be elucidated. Chemical changes can affect every stage of mRNA metabolism, encompassing splicing, maturation, translation, and degradation. (Roy, 2021). The sole changes documented for protein-coding messenger RNAs (mRNAs) are to the mRNA 5′ cap (N7-methylguanosine (m7G)), the 3′ poly(A) tail, internal inosine (I) modifications, and the conversion of internal adenosines to N6-methyladenosine (m6A) (Song & Yi, 2020). Advancements in next-generation sequencing technologies and analytical chemistry have identified numerous RNA modifications in mRNAs, although these are present at lower levels. Among the changes observed in mRNAs, m6A and pseudouridine (Ψ) are the most prevalent—mRNA vaccines for cancer. The m6A alteration is the most frequent throughout organisms, with the abundances of Ψ, N4-acetylcytidine (ac4C), Cm, and Gm nearing those of m6A (National Academies Of Sciences, E., Medicine & Committee, M. O. R. M, 2024). Conversely, 3-methylcytidine (m3C), 1-methylguanine (m1G), and 5-hydroxymethylcytidine (hm5C) are infrequent, with concentrations at least 500-fold lower than m6A, hence complicating the precise detection of these changes. Increasing evidence has demonstrated the role of m6A methylation status in embryonic development, stem cell control, adipogenesis, obesity development, type 2 diabetes pathogenesis, immunological processes, and carcinogenesis (Roy, 2021). Table 1 covers the chemical changes detected in mRNAs and their possible impacts on mRNA stability and translation.

2. mRNA-based dendritic cells (DCs) vaccines for cancer

Clinical studies have revealed that the mRNA vaccine is a groundbreaking approach for preventing and treating several diseases, including malignancies. In contrast to viral vectors or DNA vaccinations, mRNA vaccines prompt the body to synthesize proteins directly after administration. Delivery vectors and mRNAs encoding tumor antigens or immunomodulatory molecules collaborate to elicit an anti-tumor response (Tan et al., 2023). mRNA-based therapeutic cancer vaccines are well tolerated, and their intrinsic ease of production, comparable to the most effective conventional vaccine manufacturing methods, positions mRNA vaccines as a promising alternative for cancer immunotherapy. Technological advancements have enhanced the stability, structure, and delivery mechanisms of mRNA-based vaccines, and numerous clinical trials examining mRNA vaccine therapy are currently recruiting patients with diverse cancer diagnoses (Lorentzen, Haanen, Met, & Svane, 2022).

Dendritic cells (DCs) are specialized antigen-presenting cells within the immune system that can initiate or amplify anti-tumor immune responses. Consequently, dendritic cells must exhibit antigenic peptides and deliver co-stimulatory signals, such as those from CD80/CD86 and CD70, or cytokines, such as IL-12p70 (Fig. 2). An effective approach to program dendritic cells is the utilization of mRNA. mRNA is a safe, well-characterized, and secure molecule that can be readily produced with high purity. It is also cost-effective to generate and chemically well-defined, enhancing quality control and guaranteeing consistent manufacturing and

Table 1 Chemical changes and their impacts on mRNA.

Locations		Modifications	Chemical nature	Examples	Functions	References
Modification in ends mRNA's	5′ Termini	Addition of 5′ Cap	7-Methylguanosine (m7G)	M^7G Cap	Protection from degradation and assistance during translation initiation at the time of ribosomal binding	Sikorski et al. (2020)
		Methylation of adenosine nucleotide adjacent to m^7Gcap	N6-methyladenosine	m^6Am	Increase the half-life of mRNA	Wu, Pu et al. (2023)
	3′ Termini	Polyadenylation	Poly (A) Tail formation		Any defect leads to improper gene expression and controls the half-life and translation initiation process.	Joachimiak, Ciesiołka, Figura, and Fiszer (2022)
Modification in mRNA body	Noncoding regions (introns, UTRs), CDS	Inosine	Adenosine deamination at the C6 position	(I)	Functions in wobble base pairing with A, C, or U. Stability alteration.	Dutta, Deb, Sarzynska, and Lahiri (2022)
	5′ UTR, CDS, 3′ UTR	N1-Methyladenosine	Adenosine Methylation at N1 position	(m1A)	U-A Watson-Crick pairing disruption regulates mitochondrial translation.	Zhang (2019)
	5′ Cap, CDS, 3′ UTR, some 5′ UTRs	N7-Methylguanosine	Guanosine methylation at N7 position	(m7G)	Facilitates translation and provides stability to mRNA	Zhang et al. (2019)

Location	Modified nucleoside	Modification	Abbreviation	Effect	Reference
5' UTR, CDS	5-Methylcytosine	Cytosine methylation at C5 position	(m5C)	It interacts with the m5C reader protein and represses translation near the start of the codon.	Li, Wang, Zhou, Ding, and Li (2023)
tRNA, CDS of mRNA	3-Methylcytosine	Cytosine methylation at N3 position	(m3C)	Affects translation efficiency	Kleiber et al. (2022)
CDS, 3' UTR	N4-Acetylcytidine	Cytidine acetylation at N4 position	(ac4C)	Stabilizes base pairing, which enhances translation efficiency and improves tRNA decoding	Arango et al. (2018)
tRNAs, mRNAs	5-Methyluridine	Uridine methylation at the C5 position	(m5U)	Alters RNA secondary structure and ribosomal integration.	Arango et al. (2018)
CDS	2'-O-Methylation	Ribose sugar 2'-hydroxyl methylation		It helps identify self and non—self—modulates IRES-containing mRNAs.	Tang et al. (2024)
CDS	8-Oxo-7, 8-Dihydroguanosine	Guanosine oxidized form	(8-Oxo-G)	Decoding alteration, surveillance pathways triggering in mRNA, like No-go decay (NGD)	Simms and Zaher (2016)
CDS	5-Hydroxymethylcytosine	m5c oxidation by Tet family enzymes	(hm5C)	Alters mRNA's secondary structure, possibly erasing m5C effects.	Alagia and Gullerova (2022)

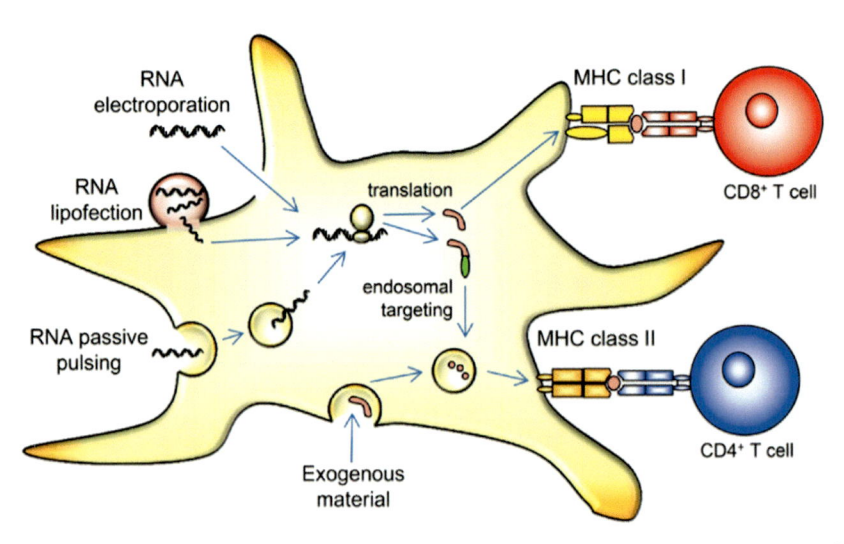

Fig. 2 DC schematic with mRNA transfection. Endocytosed and phagocytosed material is normally presented in MHC class II to CD4 + helper T cells and can cross-present in MHC class I under certain conditions. However, MHC class I primarily displays cytoplasmic proteins. Passive pulsing introduces mRNA into cells via unknown intrinsic absorption mechanisms. Electroporation or lipid reagent complexation allow it to enter the cytoplasm. A short electric pulse opens cell membrane pores, allowing RNA molecules in. The transferred mRNA is translated in the cytoplasm, presenting the encoded antigens as MHC class I. Encoding signaling and targeting sequences (green) coupled to the antigenic protein directs it to the endosomal pathway, presenting MHC class II efficiently. Figure republished by Benteyn et al. (2015), by Creative Commons Attribution (CC BY) license.

efficacy. mRNA that encodes tumor antigens and immune-modulating proteins can be effectively administered to dendritic cells to convey an anti-tumor signal. Notably, vaccines composed of mRNA-modified dendritic cells demonstrated encouraging outcomes in clinical studies (Benteyn, Heirman, Bonehill, Thielemans, & Breckpot, 2015).

Moignic *et al.* conducted a study on mRNA trimannosylated lipopolyplexes (LPR) conjugated with mannose as therapeutic cancer vaccines aimed at dendritic cells. The formulation elicited a significant local inflammatory response two days post-intradermal injection in C57BL/6 mice, subsequently leading to the recruitment and activation of dendritic cells in the associated draining lymph nodes. A significant quantity of E7-specific T cells was seen following vaccination with E7-encoded mRNA triMN-LPR. In three therapeutic pre-clinical murine tumor models—specifically E7-expressing TC1 cells, OVA-expressing EG7 cells, and

MART-1-expressing B16F0 cells—triMN-LPR containing mRNA encoding the corresponding antigens demonstrated significant curative responses in mice vaccinated seven days post initial tumor inoculation. The results demonstrate that triMN-LPR elicits an effective stimulatory immune response, facilitating therapeutic anti-cancer vaccination in mice (Le Moignic et al., 2018). Furthermore, a sialic acid (SA)-modified mRNA vaccine has been developed to concurrently achieve dendritic cell targeting along with effective endosomal/lysosomal escape. The SA modification enhanced the uptake of lipid nanoparticles (LNPs) by dendritic cells (DCs) two-fold, with over 90% of SA-modified LNPs swiftly evading early endosomes (EEs), circumventing lysosomal entry, and facilitating mRNA translation in ribosomes located in the cytoplasm and endoplasmic reticulum (ER), thereby markedly increasing the transfection efficiency of mRNA LNPs in DCs. Furthermore, cleavable PEG-lipids in mRNA vaccines were utilized, demonstrating their efficacy in enhancing cellular absorption and targeting dendritic cells. The SA-modified mRNA vaccines effectively targeted dendritic cells, demonstrating markedly better endosomal escape efficiency (90% versus 50%), enhanced tumor therapeutic efficacy, and reduced adverse effects compared to commercially available mRNA vaccines (Tang et al., 2023). Researchers has published a study on how to make mRNA-loaded LNPs work better in cells so they can be used in vaccines. The screening included a lot of different ways to control particle size as well as picking the right type of lipid and looking at its make-up. Researchers discovered that using a microfluidic device to add salt during the formation of RNA-loaded lipid nanoparticles (LNPs) can change their size to over 200 nm. The bigger LNPs delivered RNA more efficiently and in larger numbers to splenic DCs than the smaller ones. The results clearly showed a link between particle size, uptake, and gene expression activity in splenic DCs. They also showed that particles between 200 and 500 nm are the right size to target splenic DCs. It was also found that using the whole spleen to guess the transgene translation activity and the effectiveness of mRNA vaccines in splenic DCs was hard. It was found that A-11-LNP was the best formulation because it increased transgene expression and maturation in DCs and clearly fought tumors in an E.G7-OVA model compared to two other clinically useful LNP formulations (Fig. 3) (Sasaki, Sato, Okuda, Iwakawa, & Harashima, 2022). Whereas, in another investigation, the cholesterol-modified cationic peptide DP7 (VQWRIRVAVIRK) decorated on DOTAP liposomes was developed to establish a shared mRNA delivery mechanism. The system worked as a

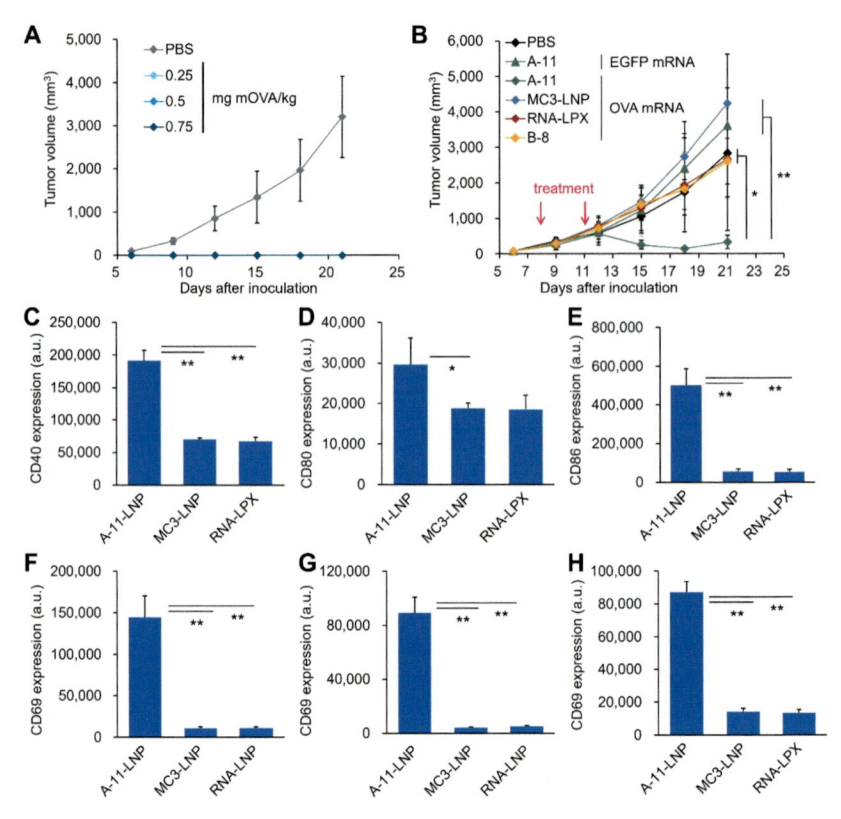

Fig. 3 Antitumor action for both prevention and treatment. (A) The A-11-LNPs' ability to prevent tumor growth in mice with E.G7-OVA tumors. The OVA mRNA-loaded A-11-LNPs administered into the veins twice, 14 and 7 days before the tumor inoculation. The amounts that were given were as shown. (B) The antitumor activity of A-11-LNPs, MC3-LNP, RNA-LPX, and B-8-LNPs. Mice with E.G7-OVA tumors were given two dose of 0.03 mg mRNA/kg of OVA-loaded formulations through the veins on days 8 and 11. In (C–E), activation markers CD40 (C), CD80 (D), and CD86 (E) were found in splenic DCs 24 h after being injected with OVA mRNA-loaded formulations at a dose of 0.03 mg mRNA/kg. In (F–H), we see how much of the activation marker CD69 is present in splenic B cells (F), T cells (G), and NK cells (H) 24 h after an IV transfer of 0.03 mg mRNA/kg of OVA loaded formulations. Figure republished from Sasaki et al. (2022), by Creative Commons License BY 4.0.

carrier and immunoadjuvant. DOTAP/DP7-C liposomes has successfully transferred mRNA into various DCs in vitro. *In vitro* and in vivo, DOTAP/DP7-C liposomes were more effective than DOTAP liposomes at stimulating DC maturation, CD103 + DC generation (antigen presentation), and proinflammatory cytokine secretion as an immunoadjuvant. In animal studies, subcutaneous administration of DOTAP/DP7-C/LL2 neoantigen-encoding mRNA complexes inhibited LL2 in situ and sub-cutaneous tumor growth and stimulated antigen-specific lymphocyte reactions superior to the group (Zhang et al., 2020).

An alternative to lipid-based mRNA delivery systems was established, utilizing poly (lactic acid) nanoparticles (PLA-NPs) and cationic cell-penetrating peptides as mRNA condensing agents. The formulations were developed in two stages: (1) the synthesis of a polyplex involving mRNAs and amphipathic cationic peptides (RALA, LAH4, or LAH4-L1), and (2) the adsorption of polyplexes onto PLA-NPs. *In vitro* results have shown that LAH4-L1/mRNA polyplexes and PLA-NP/LAH4-L1/mRNA nanocomplexes are internalized by dendritic cells through phagocytosis and clathrin-mediated endocytosis, resulting in robust protein expression in dendritic cell. They have regulated the innate immune response of dendritic cells by activating both endosomal and cytosolic Pattern Recognition Receptors (PRRs) and elicit markers of adaptive responses in primary human dendritic cells, characterized by a predominant Th1 signature. Consequently, LAH4-L1/mRNA and PLA-NP/LAH4-L1/mRNA constituted a viable framework for *ex vivo* therapy and mRNA vaccine advancement (Coolen et al., 2019). Similarly, a team of scientists has engineered a category of bioreducible lipophilic poly (beta-amino ester) nanocarriers featuring quadpolymer architecture. This platform is agnostic to the mRNA sequence, enabling one-step self-assembly for the administration of various antigen-encoding mRNAs and the co-delivery of nucleic acid-based adjuvants. An analysis of structure-function connections for NP-mediated mRNA transport to dendritic cells (DCs) revealed that a lipid subunit of the polymer structure was essential. After intravenous administration, the engineered nanoparticle design enabled targeted delivery to the spleen and selective transfection of dendritic cells without requiring surface functionalization with targeting ligands. Administration of designed nanoparticles co-delivering antigen-encoding mRNA and toll-like receptor agonist adjuvants elicited strong antigen–specific CD8 + T cell responses, culminating in effective anticancer therapy in murine in vivo models melanoma and colon adenocarcinoma (Ben-Akiva et al., 2023).

Furthermore, cationic nanoemulsions (CNEs) that were complexed with full-length tumor model antigen ovalbumin (OVA) in the form of mRNA or protein were developed and utilized as two antigenic platforms for the preparation of DCs vaccines with tailored MHC participation (known as mRNA-DCs and protein-DCs). DC vaccinations that involve both antigenic platforms have been shown to generate improved anti-tumor immunity in mouse E.G7-OVA lymphoma models and B16-OVA melanoma models. This immunity can be further enhanced by meticulously reallocating the MHC class I and II responses, as demonstrated by the studies (Shi et al., 2022).

3. mRNA delivery system

The therapeutic application of mRNA in cancer immunotherapy depends significantly on an effective delivery system to safeguard the mRNA from degradation and guarantee its arrival at the target cells (Chen, Zhu, He, & Sun, 2024). Inadequate delivery methods can result in the degradation of mRNA by nucleases or hinder its entry into target cells. Nanoparticle-based delivery systems, especially lipid-based systems, have demonstrated significant potential for effectively encapsulating and delivering mRNA, particularly in cancer treatment. These systems not only safeguard mRNA from degradation but also facilitate targeted delivery to specific tissues, thereby augmenting the therapeutic efficacy of mRNA in cancer treatment (Goyal et al., 2024; Li et al., 2022).

3.1 mRNA nanoparticle-based delivery system

3.1.1 Lipid-based mRNA delivery system

Lipid nanoparticles (LNPs) represent the most established and clinically advanced delivery systems for mRNA therapeutics. LNPs comprise ionizable lipids, cholesterol, phospholipids, and polyethylene glycol (PEG)-lipid, creating a structure that safeguards mRNA during transport and facilitates its cellular uptake. They assist in endosomal escape, enabling the release of mRNA into the cytoplasm for translation (Sharma, Babu, Jain, & Sharma, 2024). Lipid nanoparticles (LNPs) have demonstrated notable efficacy in mRNA vaccines, including those created for COVID-19, and are currently being investigated for applications in cancer immunotherapy (Thi et al., 2021). Chung et al. investigated lipid nanoparticles (LNPs) for mRNA delivery in the treatment of liver cancer. His research involved mRNA encoding an immune checkpoint inhibitor encapsulated in lipid nanoparticles, which were administered to mice with hepatic carcinoma. The LNPs enabled the introduction of mRNA into hepatic tumor cells, leading to the expression of the immune checkpoint inhibitor, which obstructed the PD-1/PD-L1 interaction. This facilitated T-cell activation, resulting in notable tumor regression and enhanced survival rates in the treated mice

(Chung, Lee, & Zhang, 2023). A first-in-human, open-label phase I study in ovarian cancer patients has recently received approval. Patients will receive intravenous vaccination before and during (neo)-adjuvant chemotherapy with a liposome-formulated mRNA vaccine (W_ova1 vaccine) that contains RNAs for three ovarian cancer tumor-associated antigens (TAAs) (ClinicalTrials.gov Identifier: NCT04163094). (Sun et al., 2023).

3.1.2 Solid lipid nanoparticles for mRNA

Solid lipid nanoparticles (SLNs) represent an alternative lipid-based delivery system. They consist of solid lipids and emulsifiers, capable of encapsulating mRNA for controlled and sustained release. Solid lipid nanoparticles (SLNs) exhibit promises for mRNA delivery owing to their capacity to preserve drug stability and enhance bioavailability. Solid lipid nanoparticles (SLNs) are increasingly recognized for their application in cancer immunotherapy due to their superior capacity to safeguard mRNA relative to conventional lipids. Solid lipid nanoparticles (SLNs) are increasingly recognized for their capacity to facilitate controlled and sustained release of therapeutic agent formulations (Hou et al., 2021; Viegas et al., 2023). A study by Mo et al. demonstrated the application of SLNs for mRNA delivery in breast cancer. The researchers encapsulated mRNA that encodes a tumor antigen within solid lipid nanoparticles, which were administered to mice with breast cancer. The SLNs efficiently safeguarded the mRNA from degradation, resulting in the successful translation of the mRNA into the target antigen within tumor cells, thereby eliciting an anti-tumor immune response and substantial tumor reduction (Mo, Kim, Choe, Shin, & Yoon, 2023). Solid lipid nanoparticles (SLNs) have been investigated for application in colorectal cancer treatment. Zhang et al. conducted a study utilizing SLNs for the delivery of mRNA that encodes a tumor-suppressing protein. The SLNs safeguarded the mRNA during transport and improved its absorption by colorectal cancer cells. Upon entering the cells, the mRNA was translated into the tumor-suppressing protein, resulting in substantial inhibition of tumor growth in the treated mice (Zhang, Ali, & Wang, 2024). A study demonstrated another application of solid lipid nanoparticles (SLNs) for mRNA delivery in lung cancer treatment. SLNs were utilized to encapsulate mRNA that encodes cytokines facilitating immune activation. In mice with lung tumors, the administration of SLNs enhanced mRNA delivery to tumor cells, prompting cytokine expression that activated an immune response against the tumor, ultimately resulting in tumor regression (Omidian, Gill, & Cubeddu, 2024).

3.1.3 Self-assembled polymeric micelles for mRNA

Polymeric micelles, created by the self-assembly of amphiphilic block copolymers, have proven to be an efficient mechanism for mRNA delivery. These micelles protect mRNA from enzymatic degradation and facilitate sustained release, enhancing the therapeutic window. The hydrophobic core of polymeric micelles encapsulates mRNA, whereas the hydrophilic shell improves biocompatibility and circulation duration. They are especially effective for administering mRNA to solid tumors in oncological treatment. Self-assembled polymeric micelles exhibit considerable potential for mRNA delivery owing to their capacity to encapsulate mRNA within their hydrophobic core, thereby safeguarding it from degradation (Ren et al., 2021; Sinani, Durgun, Cevher, & Özsoy, 2023). mRNA nanomicelles formulated with polyethylene glycol-poly(N'-(N-(2-aminoethyl)-2-aminoethyl)aspartamide) block copolymer have shown promise as viable treatments for spinal cord injury in a murine model upon the delivery of brain-derived neurotrophic factor mRNA (Crowley, Fukushima, Uchida, Kataoka, & Itaka, 2019). The administration of mRNA via micelles composed of cationic lipids and diblock polymers has demonstrated encouraging outcomes. The biodegradable micelles of DOTAP-poly(ethylene glycol)–poly(ε-caprolactone), measuring 30 nm, effectively delivered mRNA to C26 mouse colon cancer cells (60.59%) and demonstrated efficacy and safety after systemic administration for the treatment of colorectal cancer (Kakizawa, Harada, & Kataoka, 2001). Jiang et al. employed polymeric micelles for the delivery of mRNA-encoding tumor-specific antigens to glioblastoma cells. The micelles enhanced the effective absorption of mRNA by tumor cells, prompting the expression of antigens that elicited a vigorous immune response, culminating in diminished tumor size and increased survival in mouse models of glioblastoma (Melnick, Dastmalchi, Mitchell, Rahman, & Sayour, 2022). Ghasemali et al. investigated the application of polymeric micelles for the delivery of mRNA that encodes anti-angiogenic factors to solid tumors in lung cancer. The micelles effectively transported the mRNA to lung cancer cells, where it was translated into proteins that obstructed angiogenesis, the mechanism by which tumors generate new blood vessels. This led to the deprivation of nutrients for tumor cells and diminished tumor proliferation in the treated mice (Ghasemali et al., 2021).

3.1.4 Polymeric nanoparticles

Polymeric nanoparticles (PNPs) have attracted considerable attention owing to their adaptability and capacity to transport various therapeutic agents, including mRNA. These nanoparticles are generally composed of biocompatible polymers such as PLGA (poly(lactic-co-glycolic acid)) and chitosan (Misra, Patra, Varadharaj, & Verma, 2021; Neshat et al., 2023). They offer controlled release, stability, and protection for mRNA, rendering them appropriate for cancer immunotherapy applications. Polymeric nanoparticles (PNPs) are extensively utilized for mRNA delivery owing to their adaptability and capacity to transport substantial mRNA quantities (Jiang, Abedi, & Shi, 2021). Azhar et al. utilized PNPs to transport mRNA encoding a tumor suppressor gene to hepatocellular carcinoma cells. The PNPs enabled the precise delivery of mRNA, leading to the expression of the tumor suppressor protein and substantial suppression of tumor growth in a liver cancer murine model (Azhar, Bakar, Citartan, & Ahmad, 2023). A significant case pertained to the application of PNPs for mRNA delivery in prostate cancer. Researchers encapsulated mRNA encoding a cancer-testis antigen within polymeric nanoparticles, which were administered to mice with prostate cancer. The PNPs successfully transported the mRNA to tumor cells, resulting in the translation of the target antigen, which activated cytotoxic T cells and induced tumor regression (Jiang et al., 2021). PNPs have been utilized for melanoma treatment. Wang et al. developed an mRNA vaccine to combat melanoma by delivering the TRP2 tumor antigen and PD-L1-targeting siRNA using lipid-coated calcium phosphate (LCP) nanoparticles. This dual-action vaccine enhanced the immune response by activating cytotoxic T cells and downregulating PD-L1 in dendritic cells. In a mouse model, the treatment effectively inhibited tumor growth and reduced metastasis. The results highlight the potential of combining mRNA vaccines with immune checkpoint inhibition to boost antitumor immunity. This approach offers promising prospects for cancer immunotherapy (Wang, Zhang, Xu, Miao, & Huang, 2018).

3.1.5 Metallic nanoparticles

Metallic nanoparticles, especially those composed of gold and silver, provide distinctive characteristics for mRNA delivery. Their extensive surface area facilitates the binding of various functional molecules, such as mRNA, targeting ligands, and protective coatings (Soica et al., 2018). Furthermore, metallic nanoparticles can be monitored through imaging techniques, enabling real-time observation of mRNA delivery and release. A study investigated the application of gold nanoparticles for the delivery of mRNA-encoding immune checkpoint inhibitors to melanoma cells. The gold nanoparticles improved the stability and cellular absorption of mRNA, facilitating the expression of checkpoint inhibitors and stimulating an immune response that led to substantial tumor suppression (Yang et al., 2023). Silver nanoparticles were utilized for mRNA delivery in a breast cancer model. Researchers encapsulated mRNA that encodes pro-apoptotic proteins within silver nanoparticles, enabling the targeted delivery of mRNA to neoplastic cells. Upon entering the cells, the mRNA was translated into proteins that induced apoptosis, resulting in tumor reduction and enhanced survival in the treated mice (Malik, Ameta, & Mukherjee, 2023; Takáč et al., 2023). Huang et al. developed iron oxide nanoparticles (IOCCP-mRNA-PPH) to deliver mRNA into hard-to-transfect cancer cells. The nanoparticles enhanced cellular uptake, facilitated endosomal escape, and enabled efficient mRNA release, showing low toxicity. Among several formulations, IOCCP-mRNA-PPH was most effective in delivering mRNA, especially in breast, liver, and glioma cancer cells. This nanoparticle system holds promise for improved cancer treatments by optimizing mRNA delivery for gene therapies (Huang et al., 2023).

3.1.6 Silica-based nanoparticles

Silica nanoparticles (SiNPs) are inflexible, biocompatible substances that have garnered interest for their capacity to transport nucleic acids, such as mRNA. They offer a stable milieu for encapsulating mRNA, safeguarding it from enzymatic degradation, and can be functionalized with targeting ligands to enhance specificity. Silica nanoparticles provide the advantage of controlled release mechanisms, enabling the release of encapsulated mRNA to be activated by specific environmental stimuli, such as alterations in pH (Carvalho, Cordeiro, & Faneca, 2020; Tng & Low, 2023). Haddick et al. (Haddick et al., 2020) investigate the particle-size-dependent delivery of antitumoral miRNA (miR200c) using mesoporous silica nanoparticles (MSNs) targeting bladder cancer cells. MSNs, measuring between 60 and 160 nm, were functionalized with a cationic core for miRNA adsorption and capped with a block copolymer for endosomal release. The 160 nm MSN particles exhibited the greatest gene silencing efficacy, diminishing luciferase expression by 65 % in cancer cells with overexpressed EGFR. Moreover, miR200c-loaded MSNs markedly impeded cell migration and modified the cell cycle, demonstrating their potential as efficacious gene therapy vectors for cancer treatment. Dong et al. (Dong, Feng et al., 2023) focus on the design of mesoporous silica nanoparticles (MSNPs) for efficient mRNA delivery in vivo. The researchers improved mRNA complexation, stability, and delivery efficiency by modifying the MSNPs with polyethyleneimine (PEI). The optimized mRNA-PEI-MSNP system demonstrated elevated transfection rates in cellular and animal models, especially with a modified protocol that enhanced mRNA delivery efficiency. The research exhibited encouraging outcomes for mRNA-based therapies with negligible toxicity in animal models.

3.1.7 Hybrid nanoparticles

Hybrid nanoparticles amalgamate various materials, including lipids, polymers, or metals, to formulate a multifunctional delivery system. These hybrid systems are engineered to leverage the advantages of individual components while alleviating their shortcomings. Lipid-polymer hybrid nanoparticles integrate the biocompatibility and stability of polymers with the effective transfection properties of lipids. These systems provide improved mRNA stability, effective cellular uptake, and regulated release, rendering them optimal for cancer immunotherapy (Siewert et al., 2020; Zhao et al., 2018). Dong et al. investigate a novel mRNA delivery system, DMP-039, designed to augment the efficacy of cancer gene therapy. This system utilizes a hybrid nanoparticle functionalized with a peptide to enhance the delivery of mRNA encoding the suicide gene Bim. In experimental colon cancer models, the DMP-039 nanoparticle demonstrated substantial effectiveness in suppressing tumor growth and metastasis, while maintaining safety in both local and systemic administration. This research suggests that DMP-039 is a promising vehicle for mRNA-based cancer therapies (Gao et al., 2021). Moreover, the researcher investigates the application of ALKBH5 mRNA-loaded exosome-liposome hybrid nanoparticles (ELNPs) in the treatment of colorectal cancer. The hybrid nanoparticles efficiently transported mRNA into cancer cells, diminishing tumor growth and metastasis by regulating m6A methylation and triggering apoptosis. In preclinical tumor models, ALKBH5-ELNPs markedly impeded cancer progression, exhibiting safety and minimal toxicity. These findings underscore the promise of ALKBH5 mRNA-targeted nanotherapy for colorectal cancer (Wu, Yun et al., 2023).

3.1.8 Other nanoparticles

Alongside lipid-based and polymeric nanoparticles, various innovative nanoparticle systems are being engineered to improve mRNA delivery for cancer immunotherapy. These systems encompass dendrimers, silica-based nanoparticles, and hybrid nanoparticles, each providing distinct benefits for the safeguarding, targeting, and release of mRNA. These innovative platforms are especially effective in addressing the shortcomings of traditional delivery systems, including inadequate mRNA stability, suboptimal targeting, and restricted transfection efficiency (Kowalski, Rudra, Miao, & Anderson, 2019).

4. Nano-gels

Nano-gels are extensively crosslinked hydrogels capable of encapsulating mRNA, providing protection from nucleases, and facilitating targeted delivery to tumors. Their porous architecture facilitates the regulated release of mRNA, while their elevated water content enhances biocompatibility. Nano-gels have demonstrated significant potential in transporting mRNA to immune cells, rendering them effective instruments for cancer immunotherapy. Nano-gels, characterized by their highly cross-linked hydrophilic polymer networks, exhibit potential for mRNA delivery owing to their substantial water content and biocompatibility (Moscovici1, Hlevca2, Casarica1, & Pavaloiu2, 2017; Rahdar, Sayyadi, Sayyadi, & Yaghobi, 2019). Huang et al. formulated crosslinked nucleic acid nanogels for the effective delivery of mRNA to cells. The PEI-coated nanogels demonstrated increased cellular uptake and enhanced mRNA transfection efficiency in HeLa and HEK-293 cells. Various formulations of mRNA-loaded nanogels were evaluated, with the PEI-coated nanogels demonstrating superior transfection efficacy and biocompatibility. The method shows potential for efficient gene delivery in cancer treatment. (Huang et al., 2020). Duskunovic engineered cationic nanogels integrated within liposomes to facilitate the efficient delivery of mRNA to A549 cells. The nanogels demonstrated significant encapsulation efficiency and improved transfection capabilities when transporting luciferase and GFP mRNA. This system markedly enhanced mRNA delivery, leading to elevated protein expression in cells. The liposomal nanogels exhibited minimal toxicity, suggesting their promise for safe and effective gene delivery in cancer therapy (Duskunovic, Im, Lee, & Chung, 2023).

5. Dendrimers for mRNA delivery

Dendrimers are extensively branched, tree-like polymers characterized by a multitude of functional groups on their surface. This structure enables the encapsulation of mRNA molecules, preventing them from degradation

Table 2 Preclinical and clinical studies are conducted to evaluate the efficacy for cancer treatment.

Delivery systems/ approaches	Cell lines	Animal used	Mechanisms	Key findings	References
			Preclinical studies		
Poly (ethyl ethylene) phosphate liposomes with oxaliplatin	4T1 cells	C57BL/6J and BALB/c mice	Enhance antitumor immune responses in the context of OxPt-induced immunogenic cell death (ICD) by promoting dendritic cell (DC) maturation and increasing T cell infiltration.	Antigen-specific T cell respons	Yu et al. (2023)
mRNA lipid nanoparticles	HEK 293, HeLa, 4T1, and B16F10 cells	PD-1-resistant 4T1 breast cancer mice	anti-PD-1 immunotherapy	Gasdermin-mediated pyroptosis	Li, Zhang et al. (2023)
Lipid nanoparticles with 4-1BBL, OX40L, CCR7 mRNA and PAP, PSCA, PSMA, TGM4 mRNA	RM-1 cell	C57BL/6 mice	The accumulation of CD8 + T cells, specifically 4-1BB+ CD8 + T cells and OX40 + CD8 + T cells, helps suppress tumor growth and promotes the production of key immunomodulatory cytokines, including IFN-γ and TNF-α.	Enhance specific T cell cytotoxicity	Xu et al. (2024)
Combination of lipid nanoparticle–mRNA	B16F10 cells, B16F10-Luc2	C57BL/6, Batf3 -/-, and BALB/c mice	The secretion of various cytokines and chemokines, along with the upregulation of co-stimulatory	Reprogramming the tumor microenvironment	Zhang et al. (2023)

(continued)

Table 2 Preclinical and clinical studies are conducted to evaluate the efficacy for cancer treatment. (*cont'd*)

			Preclinical studies		
Delivery systems/ approaches	Cell lines	Animal used	Mechanisms	Key findings	References
formulations and dendritic cell therapy	Cells, A20 cells and 4T1 cells		molecules on dendritic cells, enhances immune activation and promotes effective antitumor responses.	and priming the T-cell responses	
EpCAM-CD3 human Fc (hFc) mRNA–lipid nanoparticles	HEK-293 cells, C30, OVCAR-5	NSG mice	Recruit natural killer (NK) cells or gamma–delta T cells to tumors by targeting specific immune cell receptors, enhancing immune surveillance and tumor destruction.	Checkpoint inhibitors, chemokines, cytokines, growth factors, and tumor microenvironment modulators regulate immune responses and influence tumor growth.	Golubovskaya et al. (2023)
Fluoroalkane-grafted polyethyleneimine polymeric nanoparticles with mRNA	DC2.4 cells and RAW264.7	C57BL/6 mic	DC maturation enhances antigen presentation, triggering effective anti-tumor immune responses.	Activate the Toll-like receptor 4 pathways	Li, Wu et al. (2023)

<table>

	Clinical trials				
Delivery systems/ approaches	Cancer (s)	Clinical trial Phase(s)	Outcomes	Experimental	NCT identifiers
PD1/PDL1/CTLA4 antibodies	Solid Tumors	Phase 1	Number of Patients with Dose Limiting Toxicity	Anti-cancer Neoantigen mRNA Vaccine	NCT06195384
targeting Epstein–Barr virus (EBV) mRNA nucleic acid	EBV-positive Advanced Malignant Tumors	Phase 1	Efficacy and safety of mRNA vaccine	Treatment Cohort	NCT05714748
Personalized mRNA Tumor Vaccine	Advanced Esophageal Cancer and Non-small Cell Lung Cancer	Not Applicable	Number of participants with treatment-related adverse events	Interventional	NCT03908671
Camrelizumab and Gemcitabine+Abraxane	Pancreatic Cancer	Early Phase 1	PD-1 inhibitor	Resectable primary pancreatic tumor	NCT06326736
Individualized mRNA neoantigen vaccine (mRNA-0523-L001)	Advanced Endocrine Tumor	Not Applicable	Maximum tolerated dose (MTD) or Dose-limiting toxicity (DLT)	mRNA-0523-L001	NCT06141369
NCI-4650 mRNA-based cancer vaccine	Colon cancer, Gastrointestinal cancer, Hepatocellular carcinoma	Phase1 and Phase 2	Number of Participants Who Had a Clinical Response (Complete Response + Partial Response) to Treatment	1/Phase – Escalating doses of mRNA vaccine 2/Phase II -MTD of mRNA vaccine established in Phase I	NCT03480152

</table>

while providing the adaptability to affix targeting ligands or other functional molecules to their surface. Dendrimers are recognized for their capacity to transport substantial quantities of mRNA and deliver them with high specificity to designated cells or tissues (Chen, Zhu, Liu, & Peng, 2022). Mbatha et al. examined dendrimer-coated gold nanoparticles (AuNPs) for effective, folate-targeted mRNA delivery in vitro. The nanoparticles, conjugated with folic acid (FA), improved transgene expression in folate receptor-positive cancer cells, including MCF-7 and KB. The FA-modified AuNPs exhibited enhanced mRNA binding, degradation protection, and improved transfection efficiency relative to non-targeted nanoparticles. Moreover, the AuNPs demonstrated biocompatibility, exhibiting low cytotoxicity and minimal apoptosis induction, thereby rendering them promising for targeted gene therapy applications (Mbatha, Maiyo, Daniels, & Singh, 2021). Zhang et al. investigated the application of ionizable amphiphilic Janus dendrimers (IAJDs) for the targeted delivery of mRNA. The dendrimers were engineered to self-assemble into nanoparticles (DNPs) capable of efficiently encapsulating and safeguarding mRNA for cellular delivery. These DNPs improved mRNA uptake and expression in both in vitro and in vivo models, exhibiting high transfection efficiency with minimal toxicity. This method demonstrates the potential for enhancing the precise delivery of mRNA in therapeutic applications, such as gene therapy and cancer treatment (Zhang et al., 2021). Xiong et al. developed theragnostic dendrimer-based lipid nanoparticles (DLNPs) incorporating PEGylated BODIPY dyes for concurrent tumor imaging and systemic mRNA delivery. These nanoparticles effectively transported mRNA and facilitated near-infrared (NIR) imaging of tumors in both in vitro and in vivo models. The DLNPs augmented mRNA synthesis in cancer cells facilitated gene expression in tumors and enabled high-contrast imaging through pH-responsive activation. This methodology demonstrates promise for prospective applications in oncology, integrating gene delivery with diagnostic imaging (Xiong, Liu, Wei, Cheng, & Siegwart, 2020).

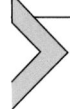

6. Preclinical and clinical trials of mRNA-based cancer therapeutics

mRNA-based cancer therapeutics are under preclinical and clinical trials. Xiao et al. (Xiao et al., 2022) address the restoration of p53 expression in hepatocellular carcinoma (HCC) to improve the efficacy of immune checkpoint blockade (ICB) therapy, whose clinical outcome is modestly achieved due to the immunosuppressive tumor microenvironment (TME). They designed CXCR4-targeting mRNA nanoparticles that potentially express p53 in HCC models. Since these nanoparticles improve anti-tumor effects when used in conjunction with anti-PD-1 therapy and reprogram the immune TME, they are superior to each monotherapy treatment. The data, therefore, indicates that the re-expression of p53 function by ICB indeed reverses the immunosuppression and stands as a considerable potential option for anti-cancer treatment. In another preclinical study by Dong et al. (Dong, Liu et al., 2023) provide a new approach to the upgrading of mRNA therapeutic in cancer therapy through the development of a method for delivery of mRNA-loaded small extracellular vesicles to the site with targeted precision. It produces sEVs loaded with IFN-γ mRNA and overexpressed CD64 on the cell surface that acts as an adaptor for trans-targeting docking by suitable targeting ligands such as anti-CD71 and anti-PD-L1 antibodies. These IMSVs preferentially target glioblastoma cells, demonstrating unprecedented anti-tumor activity in vivo, even in tumors resistant to immunotherapy in general. Such an adaptive strategy may place cancer immunotherapy at a whole new level. Some of the mRNA-based therapeutics for cancer treatment are mentioned in Table 2 with their mechanism of action and uses for the treatment of specific cancer/their cell lines.

7. Conclusions

Therapeutics mRNA presents promising approaches in cancer immunotherapy, which helps as targeted approaches to enhance the immune response, which later causes the death of cancer cells. Encoding tumor-specific antigens and immune modulators, mRNA therapies can improve the efficacy of cancer treatment. As the mRNA is unstable, it is degraded by enzymes, and lysis occurs in the cells. Due to these reasons, effective and targeted delivery systems have come to light. Several NCs are available to deliver the mRNA at the sites of cancer cells and engineer the surface of NCs. Later, it helps to target precisely the only targets cells, not the healthy cells, which improves the efficacy of NCs. Several NCs are available nowadays, such as lipid NCs, polymeric NCs, polymeric-lipids NCs, metallics NCs, hybrid NCs, etc., and scientists are continuously working on improving the precision of NCS. The mRNA-NCs or mRNA-based vaccines are in preclinical and clinical stages, which shows that mRNA-based therapies can effectively elicit strong anti-tumor responses. As the field continues to evolve, mRNA technology can potentially transform cancer treatment and concrete the way for more personalized and effective therapeutic strategies.

AI declaration

AI (ChatGPT) was used during the preparation of this chapter to improve readability and language, not to generate content.

References

Adnan, M., Afzal, O., Altamimi, A. S., Alamri, M. A., Haider, T., & Haider, M. F. (2023). Development and optimization of transethosomal gel of apigenin for topical delivery: In-vitro, ex-vivo and cell line assessment. *International Journal of Pharmaceutics, 631*, 122506.

Al Fayez, N., Nassar, M. S., Alshehri, A. A., Alnefaie, M. K., Almughem, F. A., Alshehri, B. Y., ... Tawfik, E. A. (2023). Recent advancement in mRNA vaccine development and applications. *Pharmaceutics, 15*.

Alagia, A., & Gullerova, M. (2022). The methylation game: Epigenetic and epitranscriptomic dynamics of 5-methylcytosine. *Frontiers in Cell and Developmental Biology, 10*, 915685.

Andreadis, E., Saliangas, K., Economou, A., Nikoloudis, N., Manna, I., Prodromou, K., ... Chrissidis, T. (2004). Application of radionics on primary and metastatic tumours of the liver. *Techniques in Coloproctology, 8*, s184–s186.

Arango, D., Sturgill, D., Alhusaini, N., Dillman, A. A., Sweet, T. J., Hanson, G., ... Oberdoerffer, S. (2018). Acetylation of cytidine in mRNA promotes translation efficiency. *Cell, 175*, 1872–1886.e24.

Azhar, N. A., Bakar, S. A. A., Citartan, M., & Ahmad, N. H. (2023). mRNA transcriptome profiling of human hepatocellular carcinoma cells HepG2 treated with Catharanthus roseus-silver nanoparticles. *World Journal of Hepatology, 15*, 393.

Bagchi, S., Yuan, R., & Engleman, E. G. (2021). Immune checkpoint inhibitors for the treatment of cancer: Clinical impact and mechanisms of response and resistance. *Annual Review of Pathology: Mechanisms of Disease, 16*, 223–249.

Beck, J. D., Reidenbach, D., Salomon, N., Sahin, U., Türeci, Ö., Vormehr, M., & Kranz, L. M. (2021). mRNA therapeutics in cancer immunotherapy. *Molecular Cancer, 20*, 69.

Ben-Akiva, E., Karlsson, J., Hemmati, S., Yu, H., Tzeng, S. Y., Pardoll, D. M., & Green, J. J. (2023). Biodegradable lipophilic polymeric mRNA nanoparticles for ligand-free targeting of splenic dendritic cells for cancer vaccination. *Proceedings of the National Academy of Sciences of the United States of America, 120*, e2301606120.

Benteyn, D., Heirman, C., Bonehill, A., Thielemans, K., & Breckpot, K. (2015). mRNA-based dendritic cell vaccines. *Expert Review of Vaccines, 14*, 161–176.

Cacicedo, M. L., Limeres, M. J., & Gehring, S. (2022). mRNA-based approaches to treating liver diseases. *Cells, 11*, 3328.

Carvalho, A. M., Cordeiro, R. A., & Faneca, H. (2020). Silica-based gene delivery systems: From design to therapeutic applications. *Pharmaceutics, 12*, 649.

Chahal, A., Saini, A. K., Chhillar, A. K., & Saini, R. V. (2018). Natural antioxidants as defense system against cancer. *Asian Journal of Pharmaceutical and Clinical Research*, 38–44.

Chang, X., Zhu, Z., Weng, L., Tang, X., Liu, T., Zhu, M., ... Chen, X. (2024). Selective manipulation of the mitochondria oxidative stress in different cells using intelligent mesoporous silica nanoparticles to activate on-demand immunotherapy for cancer treatment. *Small (Weinheim an der Bergstrasse, Germany), 20*, 2307310.

Chen, J., Zhu, D., Liu, X., & Peng, L. (2022). Amphiphilic dendrimer vectors for RNA delivery: State-of-the-art and future perspective. *Accounts of Materials Research, 3,* 484–497.

Chen, W., Zhu, Y., He, J., & Sun, X. (2024). Path towards mRNA delivery for cancer immunotherapy from bench to bedside. *Theranostics, 14,* 96.

Choi, S. H., Jin, S.-E., Lee, M.-K., Lim, S.-J., Park, J.-S., Kim, B.-G., ... Kim, C.-K. (2008). Novel cationic solid lipid nanoparticles enhanced p53 gene transfer to lung cancer cells. *European Journal of Pharmaceutics and Biopharmaceutics, 68,* 545–554.

Chu, D.-T., Nguyen, T. T., Tien, N. L. B., Tran, D.-K., Jeong, J.-H., Anh, P. G., ... Dinh, T. C. (2020). Recent progress of stem cell therapy in cancer treatment: molecular mechanisms and potential applications. *Cells, 9,* 563.

Chung, S., Lee, C. M., & Zhang, M. (2023). Advances in nanoparticle-based mRNA delivery for liver cancer and liver-associated infectious diseases. *Nanoscale Horizons, 8,* 10–28.

Cifuentes-Rius, A., Desai, A., Yuen, D., Johnston, A. P. R., & Voelcker, N. H. (2021). Inducing immune tolerance with dendritic cell-targeting nanomedicines. *Nature Nanotechnology, 16,* 37–46.

Coolen, A. L., Lacroix, C., Mercier-Gouy, P., Delaune, E., Monge, C., Exposito, J. Y., & Verrier, B. (2019). Poly(lactic acid) nanoparticles and cell-penetrating peptide potentiate mRNA-based vaccine expression in dendritic cells triggering their activation. *Biomaterials, 195,* 23–37.

Crowley, S. T., Fukushima, Y., Uchida, S., Kataoka, K., & Itaka, K. (2019). Enhancement of motor function recovery after spinal cord injury in mice by delivery of brain-derived neurotrophic factor mRNA. *Molecular Therapy-Nucleic Acids, 17,* 465–476.

De Baere, T., & Deschamps, F. (2014). New tumor ablation techniques for cancer treatment (microwave, electroporation). *Diagnostic and Interventional Imaging, 95,* 677–682.

Debela, D. T., Muzazu, S. G., Heraro, K. D., Ndalama, M. T., Mesele, B. W., Haile, D. C., ... Manyazewal, T. (2021). New approaches and procedures for cancer treatment: Current perspectives. *SAGE Open Medicine, 9,* 20503121211034366.

Delgado, M., & Garcia-Sanz, J. A. (2023). Therapeutic monoclonal antibodies against cancer: Present and future. *Cells, 12,* 2837.

Dong, S., Feng, Z., Ma, R., Zhang, T., Jiang, J., Li, Y., ... Liu, X. (2023). Engineered design of a mesoporous silica nanoparticle-based nanocarrier for efficient mRNA delivery in vivo. *Nano Letters, 23,* 2137–2147.

Dong, S., Liu, X., Bi, Y., Wang, Y., Antony, A., Lee, D., ... Jiang, W. (2023). Adaptive design of mRNA-loaded extracellular vesicles for targeted immunotherapy of cancer. *Nature Communications, 14,* 6610.

Duskunovic, N., Im, S. H., Lee, J., & Chung, H. J. (2023). Effective mRNA delivery by condensation with cationic nanogels incorporated into liposomes. *Molecular Pharmaceutics, 20,* 3088–3099.

Dutta, N., Deb, I., Sarzynska, J., & Lahiri, A. (2022). Inosine and its methyl derivatives: Occurrence, biogenesis, and function in RNA. *Progress in Biophysics and Molecular Biology, 169,* 21–52.

Eisenhut, P., Marx, N., Borsi, G., Papež, M., Ruggeri, C., Baumann, M., & Borth, N. (2023). Manipulating gene expression levels in mammalian cell factories: An outline of synthetic molecular toolboxes to achieve multiplexed control. *New Biotechnology.*

Ellis, G. I., Sheppard, N. C., & Riley, J. L. (2021). Genetic engineering of T cells for immunotherapy. *Nature Reviews. Genetics, 22,* 427–447.

Gao, Y., Men, K., Pan, C., Li, J., Wu, J., Chen, X., ... Duan, X. (2021). Functionalized DMP-039 hybrid nanoparticle as a novel mRNA vector for efficient cancer suicide gene therapy. *International Journal of Nanomedicine,* 5211–5232.

Ghasemali, S., Farajnia, S., Barzegar, A., Rahmati-Yamchi, M., Baghban, R., Rahbarnia, L., & Nodeh, H. R. (2021). New developments in anti-angiogenic therapy of cancer, review and update. *Anti-Cancer Agents in Medicinal Chemistry (Formerly Current Medicinal Chemistry-Anti-Cancer Agents), 21*, 3–19.

Golubovskaya, V., Sienkiewicz, J., Sun, J., Huang, Y., Hu, L., Zhou, H., ... Wu, L. (2023). mRNA-lipid nanoparticle (LNP) delivery of humanized EpCAM-CD3 bispecific antibody significantly blocks colorectal cancer tumor growth. *Cancers [Online], 15.*

Goyal, F., Chattopadhyay, A., Navik, U., Jain, A., Reddy, P. H., Bhatti, G. K., & Bhatti, J. S. (2024). Advancing cancer immunotherapy: The potential of mRNA vaccines as a promising therapeutic approach. *Advanced Therapeutics, 7*, 2300255.

Gupta, I., Hussein, O., Sastry, K. S., Bougarn, S., Gopinath, N., Chin-Smith, E., ... Maccalli, C. (2023). Deciphering the complexities of cancer cell immune evasion: Mechanisms and therapeutic implications. *Advances in Cancer Biology–Metastasis, 8*, 100107.

Haddick, L., Zhang, W., Reinhard, S., Möller, K., Engelke, H., Wagner, E., & Bein, T. (2020). Particle-size-dependent delivery of antitumoral miRNA using targeted mesoporous silica nanoparticles. *Pharmaceutics, 12*, 505.

Haider, T., Pandey, V., Banjare, N., Gupta, P. N., & Soni, V. (2020). Drug resistance in cancer: Mechanisms and tackling strategies. *Pharmacological Reports: PR, 72*, 1125–1151.

Haider, T., Pandey, V., Behera, C., Kumar, P., Gupta, P. N., & Soni, V. (2020). Spectrin conjugated PLGA nanoparticles for potential membrane phospholipid interactions: Development, optimization and in vitro studies. *Journal of Drug Delivery Science and Technology, 60*, 102087.

Haider, T., Pandey, V., Sandha, K. K., Gupta, P. N., & Soni, V. (2020). Implication of nanomedicine in therapy of oxidative stress induced cancer. *Handbook of Oxidative Stress in Cancer: Mechanistic Aspects*, 1–21.

Haider, T., Pandey, V., Behera, C., Kumar, P., Gupta, P. N., & Soni, V. (2022). Nisin and nisin-loaded nanoparticles: A cytotoxicity investigation. *Drug Development and Industrial Pharmacy, 48*, 310–321.

Haider, T., & Soni, V. (2022). Response surface methodology and artificial neural network-based modeling and optimization of phosphatidylserine targeted nanocarriers for effective treatment of cancer: In vitro and in silico studies. *Journal of Drug Delivery Science and Technology, 75*, 103663.

Haider, T., Tiwari, R., Vyas, S. P., & Soni, V. (2019). Molecular determinants as therapeutic targets in cancer chemotherapy: An update. *Pharmacology & Therapeutics, 200*, 85–109.

Hinnebusch, A. G., Ivanov, I. P., & Sonenberg, N. (2016). Translational control by 5′-untranslated regions of eukaryotic mRNAs. *Science (New York, N. Y.), 352*, 1413–1416.

Hosseinkhani, H., Domb, A. J., Sharifzadeh, G., & Nahum, V. (2023). Gene therapy for regenerative medicine. *Pharmaceutics, 15.*

Hou, X., Zaks, T., Langer, R., & Dong, Y. (2021). Lipid nanoparticles for mRNA delivery. *Nature Reviews Materials, 6*, 1078–1094.

Huang, J., Lin, G., Juenke, T., Chung, S., Lai, N., Zhang, T., ... Zhang, M. (2023). Iron oxide nanoparticle-mediated mRNA delivery to hard-to-transfect cancer cells. *Pharmaceutics, 15*, 1946.

Huang, X., Zheng, R., Ding, F., Yang, J., Xie, M., Liu, X., ... Zhang, C. (2020). Efficient delivery of mRNA using crosslinked nucleic acid nanogel as a carrier. *ACS Materials Letters, 2*, 1509–1515.

Hussain, A., Yang, H., Zhang, M., Liu, Q., Alotaibi, G., Irfan, M., ... Huang, Y. (2022). mRNA vaccines for COVID-19 and diverse diseases. *Journal of Controlled Release: Official Journal of the Controlled Release Society, 345*, 314–333.

Jana, D., He, B., Chen, Y., Liu, J., & Zhao, Y. (2024). A defect-engineered nanozyme for targeted NIR-II photothermal immunotherapy of cancer. *Advanced Materials, 36*, 2206401.

Jiang, X., Abedi, K., & Shi, J. (2021). Polymeric nanoparticles for RNA delivery. *Reference Module in Materials Science and Materials Engineering.*

Joachimiak, P., Ciesiołka, A., Figura, G., & Fiszer, A. (2022). Implications of Poly (A) tail processing in repeat expansion diseases. *Cells, 11*, 677.

Kakizawa, Y., Harada, A., & Kataoka, K. (2001). Glutathione-sensitive stabilization of block copolymer micelles composed of antisense DNA and thiolated poly (ethylene glycol)-b lock–poly (l-lysine): A potential carrier for systemic delivery of antisense DNA. *Biomacromolecules, 2*, 491–497.

Kleiber, N., Lemus-Diaz, N., Stiller, C., Heinrichs, M., Mai, M. M.-Q., Hackert, P., ... Bohnsack, M. T. (2022). The RNA methyltransferase METTL8 installs m3C32 in mitochondrial tRNAsThr/Ser(UCN) to optimise tRNA structure and mitochondrial translation. *Nature Communications, 13*, 209.

Kowalski, P. S., Rudra, A., Miao, L., & Anderson, D. G. (2019). Delivering the messenger: Advances in technologies for therapeutic mRNA delivery. *Molecular Therapy, 27*, 710–728.

Le Moignic, A., Malard, V., Benvegnu, T., Lemiègre, L., Berchel, M., Jaffrès, P. A., ... Mateo, V. (2018). Preclinical evaluation of mRNA trimannosylated lipopolyplexes as therapeutic cancer vaccines targeting dendritic cells. *Journal of Controlled Release, 278*, 110–121.

Li, D. F., Liu, Q. S., Yang, M. F., Xu, H. M., Zhu, M. Z., Zhang, Y., ... Wang, L. S. (2023). Nanomaterials for mRNA-based therapeutics: Challenges and opportunities. *Bioengineering & Translational Medicine, 8*, e10492.

Li, F., Zhang, X.-Q., Ho, W., Tang, M., Li, Z., Bu, L., & Xu, X. (2023). mRNA lipid nanoparticle-mediated pyroptosis sensitizes immunologically cold tumors to checkpoint immunotherapy. *Nature Communications, 14*, 4223.

Li, J., Wu, Y., Xiang, J., Wang, H., Zhuang, Q., Wei, T., ... Peng, R. (2023). Fluoroalkane modified cationic polymers for personalized mRNA cancer vaccines. *Chemical Engineering Journal, 456*, 140930.

Li, P., Wang, W., Zhou, R., Ding, Y., & Li, X. (2023). The m(5) C methyltransferase NSUN2 promotes codon-dependent oncogenic translation by stabilising tRNA in anaplastic thyroid cancer. *Clinical and Translational Medicine, 13*, e1466.

Li, Y., Wang, M., Peng, X., Yang, Y., Chen, Q., Liu, J., ... Li, X. (2023). mRNA vaccine in cancer therapy: Current advance and future outlook. *Clinical and Translational Medicine, 13*, e1384.

Li, M., Li, Y., Li, S., Jia, L., Wang, H., Li, M., ... Li, W. (2022). The nano delivery systems and applications of mRNA. *European Journal of Medicinal Chemistry, 227*, 113910.

Licatalosi, D. D., & Darnell, R. B. (2010). RNA processing and its regulation: Global insights into biological networks. *Nature Reviews. Genetics, 11*, 75–87.

Lorentzen, C. L., Haanen, J. B., Met, Ö., & Svane, I. M. (2022). Clinical advances and ongoing trials on mRNA vaccines for cancer treatment. *The Lancet Oncology, 23*, e450–e458.

Luo, L., Wang, H., Tian, W., Li, X., Zhu, Z., Huang, R., & Luo, H. (2021). Targeting ferroptosis-based cancer therapy using nanomaterials: Strategies and applications. *Theranostics, 11*, 9937.

Malik, P., Ameta, R. K., & Mukherjee, T. K. (2023). *Emerging drug delivery potential of gold and silver nanoparticles to lung and breast cancers. Practical approach to mammalian cell and organ culture.* Springer.

Mavi, A. K., Gaur, S., Gaur, G., Babita, Kumar, N., & Kumar, U. (2023). CAR T-cell therapy: Reprogramming patient's immune cell to treat cancer. *Cellular Signalling, 105*, 110638.

Mayr, C. (2017). Regulation by 3′-untranslated regions. *Annual Review of Genetics, 51*, 171–194.

Mayr, C. (2019). What are 3′ UTRs doing? *Cold Spring Harbor Perspectives in Biology, 11*, a034728.

Mbatha, L. S., Maiyo, F., Daniels, A., & Singh, M. (2021). Dendrimer-coated gold nanoparticles for efficient folate-targeted mRNA delivery in vitro. *Pharmaceutics, 13*, 900.

Mchale, A. P., Callan, J. F., Nomikou, N., Fowley, C., & Callan, B. (2016). Sonodynamic therapy: Concept, mechanism and application to cancer treatment. *Therapeutic Ultrasound, 429*–450.

Melnick, K., Dastmalchi, F., Mitchell, D., Rahman, M., & Sayour, E. J. (2022). Contemporary RNA therapeutics for glioblastoma. *Neuromolecular Medicine, 24*, 8–12.

Misra, R., Patra, B., Varadharaj, S., & Verma, R. S. (2021). Establishing the promising role of novel combination of triple therapeutics delivery using polymeric nanoparticles for Triple negative breast cancer therapy. *BioImpacts: BI, 11*, 199.

Mo, K., Kim, A., Choe, S., Shin, M., & Yoon, H. (2023). Overview of solid lipid nanoparticles in breast cancer therapy. *Pharmaceutics, 15*, 2065.

Moscovici1, M., Hlevca2, C., Casarica1, A., & Pavaloiu2, R. D. (2017). Nanocellulose and nanogels as modern drug delivery systems. *Nanocellulose and Nanohydrogel Matrices: Biotechnological and Biomedical Applications, 209*–269.

Kuhn, N., Beissert, A., Simon, T., Vallazza, P., Buck, B., Davies, J. P., ... Sahin, U. (2012). mRNA as a versatile tool for exogenous protein expression. *Current Gene Therapy, 12*, 347–361.

National Academies Of Sciences, E., Medicine & Committee, M. O. R. M. (2024). Ideation challenge commissioned papers. Charting a future for sequencing RNA and its modifications: A new era for biology and medicine. National Academies Press (US).

Neshat, S. Y., Chan, C. H. R., Harris, J., Zmily, O. M., Est-Witte, S., Karlsson, J., ... Green, J. J. (2023). Polymeric nanoparticle gel for intracellular mRNA delivery and immunological reprogramming of tumors. *Biomaterials, 300*, 122185.

Omidian, H., Gill, E. J., & Cubeddu, L. X. (2024). Lipid nanoparticles in lung cancer therapy. *Pharmaceutics, 16*, 644.

Palucka, K., & Banchereau, J. (2012). Cancer immunotherapy via dendritic cells. *Nature Reviews. Cancer, 12*, 265–277.

Pandey, P. R., Young, K. H., Kumar, D., & Jain, N. (2022). RNA-mediated immunotherapy regulating tumor immune microenvironment: Next wave of cancer therapeutics. *Molecular Cancer, 21*, 58.

Pandey, V., Haider, T., Chandak, A. R., Chakraborty, A., Banerjee, S., & Soni, V. (2020). Surface modified silk fibroin nanoparticles for improved delivery of doxorubicin: Development, characterization, in-vitro studies. *International Journal of Biological Macromolecules, 164*, 2018–2027.

Pandey, V., Haider, T., Gour, V., Soni, V., & Gupta, P. N. (2020). *Prodrugs in cancer nanomedicine and therapy. Recent advancement in prodrugs*. CRC Press.

Passmore, L. A., & Coller, J. (2022). Roles of mRNA poly (A) tails in regulation of eukaryotic gene expression. *Nature Reviews. Molecular Cell Biology, 23*, 93–106.

Propper, D. J., & Balkwill, F. R. (2022). Harnessing cytokines and chemokines for cancer therapy. *Nature Reviews Clinical Oncology, 19*, 237–253.

Qin, S., Tang, X., Chen, Y., Chen, K., Fan, N., Xiao, W., ... Wu, M. (2022). mRNA-based therapeutics: Powerful and versatile tools to combat diseases. *Signal Transduction and Targeted Therapy, 7*, 166.

Rahdar, A., Sayyadi, K., Sayyadi, J., & Yaghobi, Z. (2019). Nano-gels: A versatile nanocarrier platform for drug delivery systems: A mini review. *Nanomedicine Research Journal, 4*, 1–9.

Ramachandran, S., Satapathy, S. R., & Dutta, T. (2022). Delivery strategies for mRNA Vaccines. *Pharmaceutical Medicine, 36*, 11–20.

Ren, J., Cao, Y., Li, L., Wang, X., Lu, H., Yang, J., & Wang, S. (2021). Self-assembled polymeric micelle as a novel mRNA delivery carrier. *Journal of Controlled Release, 338*, 537–547.

Roy, B. (2021). Effects of mRNA modifications on translation: An overview. *RNA Modifications: Methods and Protocols,* 327–356.

Sahin, U., Karikó, K., & Türeci, Ö. (2014). mRNA-based therapeutics—Developing a new class of drugs. *Nature Reviews. Drug Discovery, 13*, 759–780.

Sasaki, K., Sato, Y., Okuda, K., Iwakawa, K., & Harashima, H. (2022). mRNA-loaded lipid nanoparticles targeting dendritic cells for cancer immunotherapy. *Pharmaceutics, 14.*

Saxena, M., Van Der Burg, S. H., Melief, C. J., & Bhardwaj, N. (2021). Therapeutic cancer vaccines. *Nature Reviews. Cancer, 21*, 360–378.

Mature mRNA [Online]. < Available: https://theory.labster.com/mrna-maduration/ > [Accessed 22/09/2024].

Scitable. Poly-A tail [Online]. Natue Education. Available: https://www.nature.com/scitable/definition/poly-a-tail-276/#:~:text=The%20poly%2DA%20tail%20is,modifications%20known%20as%20RNA%20processing. [Accessed 22/09/2024].

Sharma, T., Babu, M. A., Jain, A., & Sharma, D. (2024). Lipid-based nanocarriers for mRNA delivery: Vital considerations and applications. *Nanoscience & Nanotechnology-Asia, 14*, 49–61.

Shchelochkov, O.A. (2024). Open reading frame [Online]. National Human Genome Research Institute. Avialble < https://www.genome.gov/genetics-glossary/Open-Reading-Frame >. [Accessed on: 22 Nov. 2024].

Shi, Y., Liu, Y., Huang, J., Luo, Z., Guo, X., Jiang, M., ... You, J. (2022). Optimized mobilization of MHC class I- and II- restricted immunity by dendritic cell vaccine potentiates cancer therapy. *Theranostics, 12*, 3488–3502.

Siewert, C. D., Haas, H., Cornet, V., Nogueira, S. S., Nawroth, T., Uebbing, L., ... Schroer, M. A. (2020). Hybrid biopolymer and lipid nanoparticles with improved transfection efficacy for mRNA. *Cells, 9*, 2034.

Sikorski, P. J., Warminski, M., Kubacka, D., Ratajczak, T., Nowis, D., Kowalska, J., & Jemielity, J. (2020). The identity and methylation status of the first transcribed nucleotide in eukaryotic mRNA 5′ cap modulates protein expression in living cells. *Nucleic Acids Research, 48*, 1607–1626.

Simms, C. L., & Zaher, H. S. (2016). Quality control of chemically damaged RNA. *Cellular and Molecular Life Sciences: CMLS, 73*, 3639–3653.

Sinani, G., Durgun, M. E., Cevher, E., & Özsoy, Y. (2023). Polymeric-micelle-based delivery systems for nucleic acids. *Pharmaceutics, 15*, 2021.

Singhai, M., Pandey, V., Ashique, S., Gupta, G. D., Arora, D., Haider, T., & Mishra, N. (2023). Design and evaluation of SLNs encapsulated curcumin-based topical formulation for the management of cervical cancer. *Anti-Cancer Agents in Medicinal Chemistry (Formerly Current Medicinal Chemistry-Anti-Cancer Agents), 23*, 1866–1879.

Soica, C., Pinzaru, I., Trandafirescu, C., Andrica, F., Danciu, C., Mioc, M., ... Dehelean, C. (2018). *Silver-, gold-, and iron-based metallic nanoparticles: Biomedical applications as theranostic agents for cancer. Design of nanostructures for theranostics applications.* Elsevier.

Song, J., & Yi, C. (2020). Reading chemical modifications in the transcriptome. *Journal of Molecular Biology, 432*, 1824–1839.

Spurna, Z., Capkova, P., Srovnal, J., Duchoslavova, J., Punova, L., Aleksijevic, D., & Vrtel, R. (2022). Clinical impact of variants in non-coding regions of SHOX–current knowledge. *Gene, 818*, 146238.

Sun, H., Zhang, Y., Wang, G., Yang, W., & Xu, Y. (2023). mRNA-based therapeutics in cancer treatment. *Pharmaceutics, 15*, 622.

Takáč, P., Michalková, R., Čižmáriková, M., Bedlovičová, Z., Balážová, Ľ., & Takáčová, G. (2023). The role of silver nanoparticles in the diagnosis and treatment of cancer: Are there any perspectives for the future? *Life (Chicago, Ill.: 1978), 13*, 466.

Takara. 5-prime capping of mRNA [Online]. Available: https://www.takarabio.com/learning-centers/mrna-and-cdna-synthesis/mrna-synthesis/5-prime-capping-of-mrna [Accessed 22/09/2024].

Tan, T., Deng, S. T., Wu, B. H., Yang, Q., Wu, M. W., Wu, H., ... Xu, C. (2023). mRNA vaccine – A new cancer treatment strategy. *Current Cancer Drug Targets, 23*, 669–681.

Tang, X., Zhang, J., Sui, D., Yang, Q., Wang, T., Xu, Z., ... Deng, Y. (2023). Simultaneous dendritic cells targeting and effective endosomal escape enhance sialic acid-modified mRNA vaccine efficacy and reduce side effects. *Journal of Controlled Release: Official Journal of the Controlled Release Society, 364*, 529–545.

Tang, Y., Wu, Y., Wang, S., Lu, X., Gu, X., Li, Y., ... Chen, Q. (2024). An integrative platform for detection of RNA 2′-O-methylation reveals its broad distribution on mRNA. *Cell Reports Methods, 4*, 100721.

Thi, T. T. H., Suys, E. J., Lee, J. S., Nguyen, D. H., Park, K. D., & Truong, N. P. (2021). Lipid-based nanoparticles in the clinic and clinical trials: From cancer nanomedicine to COVID-19 vaccines. *Vaccines, 9*, 359.

Tng, D. J. H., & Low, J. G. H. (2023). Current status of silica-based nanoparticles as therapeutics and its potential as therapies against viruses. *Antiviral Research, 210*, 105488.

Viegas, C., Patrício, A. B., Prata, J. M., Nadhman, A., Chintamaneni, P. K., & Fonte, P. (2023). Solid lipid nanoparticles vs. nanostructured lipid carriers: A comparative review. *Pharmaceutics, 15*, 1593.

Vishwakarma, M., Haider, T., & Soni, V. (2024). Next-generation skin cancer treatment: A quality by design perspective on artificial neural network-optimized cationic ethosomes with bleomycin sulphate. *Journal of Drug Delivery Science and Technology, 96*, 105705.

Wadhwa, A., Aljabbari, A., Lokras, A., Foged, C., & Thakur, A. (2020). Opportunities and challenges in the delivery of mRNA-based vaccines. *Pharmaceutics, 12*.

Wang, X., Zhong, X., Liu, Z., & Cheng, L. (2020). Recent progress of chemodynamic therapy-induced combination cancer therapy. *Nano Today, 35*, 100946.

Wang, Y., Zhang, L., Xu, Z., Miao, L., & Huang, L. (2018). mRNA vaccine with antigen-specific checkpoint blockade induces an enhanced immune response against established melanoma. *Molecular Therapy, 26*, 420–434.

Wang, Y., Zhang, Z., Luo, J., Han, X., Wei, Y., & Wei, X. (2021). mRNA vaccine: A potential therapeutic strategy. *Molecular Cancer, 20*, 33.

Who, I. (2024). *WHO News release. Global cancer burden growing, amidst mounting need for services*. World health Organisation.

Wu, S., Yun, J., Tang, W., Familiari, G., Relucenti, M., Wu, J., ... Chen, R. (2023). Therapeutic m6A eraser ALKBH5 mRNA-loaded exosome–liposome hybrid nanoparticles inhibit progression of colorectal cancer in preclinical tumor models. *ACS Nano, 17*, 11838–11854.

Wu, Y., Pu, X., Wu, S., Zhang, Y., Fu, S., Tang, H., ... Xu, M. (2023). PCIF1, the only methyltransferase of N6, 2-O-dimethyladenosine. *Cancer Cell International, 23*, 226.

Xiao, Y., Chen, J., Zhou, H., Zeng, X., Ruan, Z., Pu, Z., ... Shi, J. (2022). Combining p53 mRNA nanotherapy with immune checkpoint blockade reprograms the immune microenvironment for effective cancer therapy. *Nature Communications, 13*, 758.

Xiong, H., Liu, S., Wei, T., Cheng, Q., & Siegwart, D. J. (2020). Theranostic dendrimer-based lipid nanoparticles containing PEGylated BODIPY dyes for tumor imaging and systemic mRNA delivery in vivo. *Journal of Controlled Release, 325*, 198–205.

Xu, Z., Xiao, Z.-X., Wang, J., Qiu, H.-W., Cao, F., Zhang, S.-Q., ... Pang, J. (2024). Novel mRNA adjuvant ImmunER enhances prostate cancer tumor-associated antigen mRNA therapy via augmenting T cell activity. *OncoImmunology, 13*, 2373526.

Yang, B., Gao, J., Pei, Q., Xu, H., & Yu, H. (2020). Engineering prodrug nanomedicine for cancer immunotherapy. *Advanced Science, 7*, 2002365.

Yang, W., Cao, J., Cheng, H., Chen, L., Yu, M., Chen, Y., & Cui, X. (2023). Nanoformulations targeting immune cells for cancer therapy: mRNA therapeutics. *Bioactive Materials, 23*, 438–470.

Yap, T. A., Parkes, E. E., Peng, W., Moyers, J. T., Curran, M. A., & Tawbi, H. A. (2021). Development of immunotherapy combination strategies in cancer. *Cancer discovery, 11*, 1368–1397.

You, K., Wang, Q., Osman, M. S., Kim, D., Li, Q., Feng, C., ... Yang, K. (2024). Advanced strategies for combinational immunotherapy of cancer based on polymeric nanomedicines. *BMEMat*, e12067.

Yu, X., Li, H., Dong, C., Qi, S., Yang, K., Bai, B., ... Yu, G. (2023). Poly(ethyl ethylene phosphate): Overcoming the "polyethylene glycol dilemma" for cancer immunotherapy and mRNA vaccination. *ACS Nano, 17*, 23814–23828.

Zhang, D., Atochina-Vasserman, E. N., Maurya, D. S., Liu, M., Xiao, Q., Lu, J., ... Ni, H. (2021). Targeted delivery of mRNA with one-component ionizable amphiphilic Janus dendrimers. *Journal of the American Chemical Society, 143*, 17975–17982.

Zhang, J., Ali, K., & Wang, J. (2024). Research advances of lipid nanoparticles in the treatment of colorectal cancer. *International Journal of Nanomedicine*, 6693–6715.

Zhang, L.-S., Liu, C., Ma, H., Dai, Q., Sun, H.-L., Luo, G., ... Dong, X. (2019). Transcriptome-wide mapping of internal N7-methylguanosine methylome in mammalian mRNA. *Molecular Cell, 74*, 1304–1316 e8.

Zhang, L. (2019). *High-Resolution Mapping of mRNA Modifications*.

Zhang, R., Tang, L., Tian, Y., Ji, X., Hu, Q., Zhou, B., ... Yang, L. (2020). DP7-C-modified liposomes enhance immune responses and the antitumor effect of a neoantigen-based mRNA vaccine. *Journal of Controlled Release, 328*, 210–221.

Zhang, Y., Hou, X., Du, S., Xue, Y., Yan, J., Kang, D. D., ... Dong, Y. (2023). Close the cancer-immunity cycle by integrating lipid nanoparticle-mRNA formulations and dendritic cell therapy. *Nature Nanotechnology, 18*, 1364–1374.

Zhao, W., Zhang, C., Li, B., Zhang, X., Luo, X., Zeng, C., ... Dong, Y. (2018). Lipid polymer hybrid nanomaterials for mRNA delivery. *Cellular and Molecular Bioengineering, 11*, 397–406.

Printed in the United States
by Baker & Taylor Publisher Services